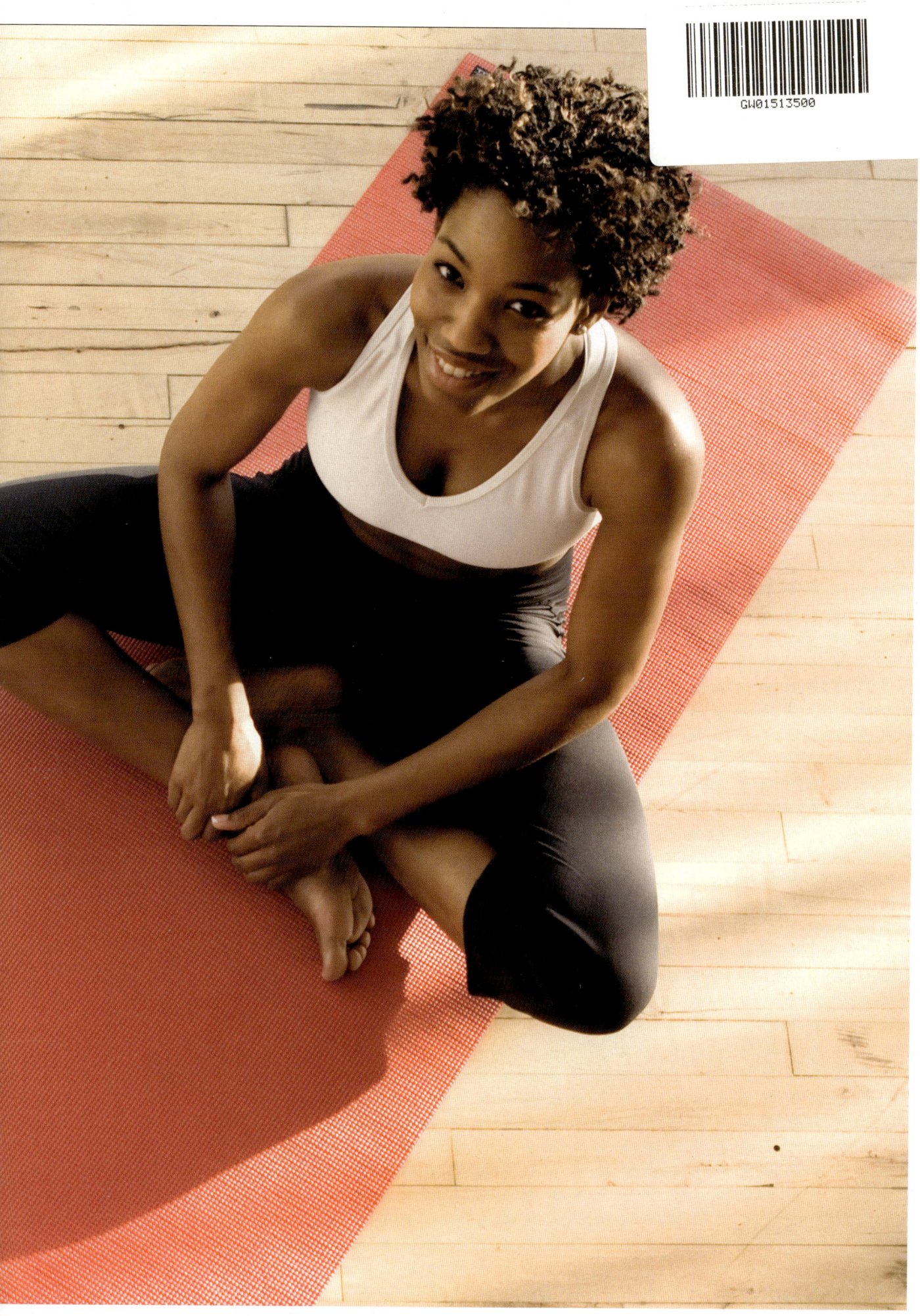

FUTURE

10-minute morning YOGA

Future PLC Quay House, The Ambury, Bath, BA1 1UA

Editorial
Editor **Mary Comber**
Art Editor **Kelly Flood**
Chief Sub-Editor **Sheila Reid**
Compiled by **Alice Pattillo & Lora Barnes**
Senior Art Editor **Andy Downes**
Head of Art & Design **Greg Whitaker**
Editorial Director **Jon White**

Cover images
Danny Bird

Photography
Danny Bird
All copyrights and trademarks are recognised and respected
Retouching **Colin Beagley**
Hair & make-up **Lisa Waite** (@lisawaitemakeup)
Yoga model **Zoe Thresher at WModel**
Yoga instruction **Aki Omori**

Advertising
Media packs are available on request
Commercial Director **Clare Dove**

International
Head of Print Licensing **Rachel Shaw**
licensing@futurenet.com
www.futurecontenthub.com

Circulation
Head of Newstrade **Tim Mathers**

Production
Head of Production **Mark Constance**
Production Project Manager **Matthew Eglinton**
Advertising Production Manager **Joanne Crosby**
Digital Editions Controller **Jason Hudson**
Production Managers **Keely Miller, Nola Cokely, Vivienne Calvert, Fran Twentyman**

Printed in the UK
Distributed by Marketforce, 5 Churchill Place, Canary Wharf, London, E14 5HU www.marketforce.co.uk – For enquiries, please email: mfcommunications@futurenet.com

10-Minute Morning Yoga Second Edition (LBZ5258)
© 2023 Future Publishing Limited

We are committed to only using magazine paper which is derived from responsibly managed, certified forestry and chlorine-free manufacture. The paper in this bookazine was sourced and produced from sustainable managed forests, conforming to strict environmental and socioeconomic standards.

All contents © 2023 Future Publishing Limited or published under licence. All rights reserved. No part of this magazine may be used, stored, transmitted or reproduced in any way without the prior written permission of the publisher. Future Publishing Limited (company number 2008885) is registered in England and Wales. Registered office: Quay House, The Ambury, Bath BA1 1UA. All information contained in this publication is for information only and is, as far as we are aware, correct at the time of going to press. Future cannot accept any responsibility for errors or inaccuracies in such information. You are advised to contact manufacturers and retailers directly with regard to the price of products/services referred to in this publication. Apps and websites mentioned in this publication are not under our control. We are not responsible for their contents or any other changes or updates to them. This magazine is fully independent and not affiliated in any way with the companies mentioned herein.

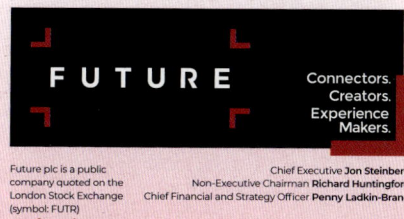

Future plc is a public company quoted on the London Stock Exchange (symbol: FUTR)
www.futureplc.com

Chief Executive **Jon Steinberg**
Non-Executive Chairman **Richard Huntingford**
Chief Financial and Strategy Officer **Penny Ladkin-Brand**

Tel +44 (0)1225 442 244

 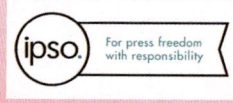

CONTENTS

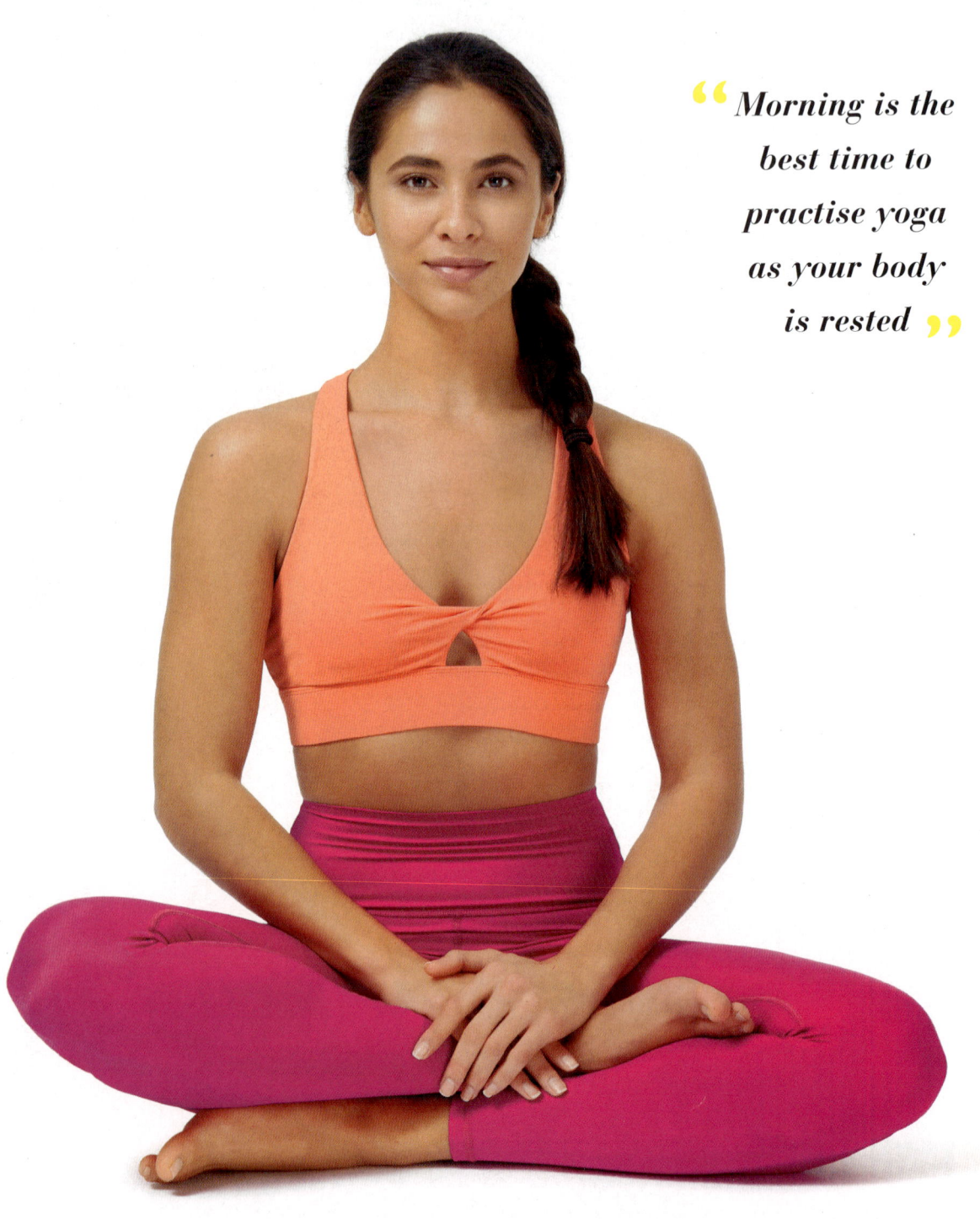

" *Morning is the best time to practise yoga as your body is rested* "

Contents

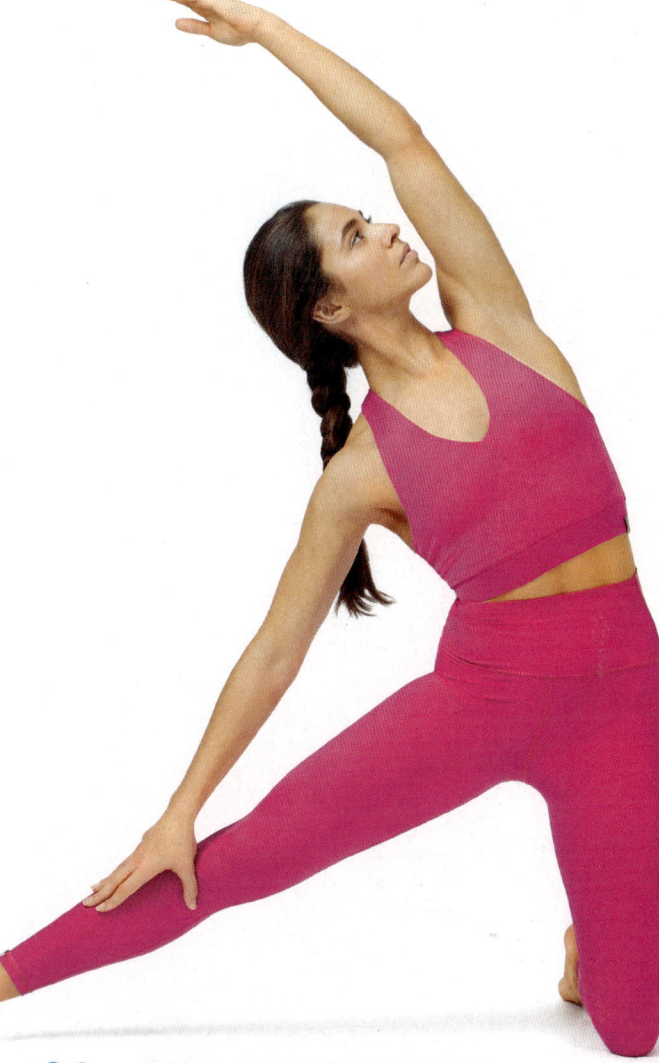

8	How to use this book
10	Introduction
12	The benefits
22	The magic of morning yoga
24	How to be an early bird

26 THE BASICS
- **28** Breathing basics
- **30** Perfect posture
- **32** Tips for morning yoga
- **34** Your yoga kit

38 THE POSTURES
- **40** Standing poses
- **72** Backbend poses
- **82** Sitting poses
- **88** Reclining poses

94 THE SEQUENCES
- **96** Warm-up
- **102** Sun salutations
- **108** Energise your day
- **110** Ground yourself
- **112** Find your focus
- **114** Morning stretch

116 TAKE IT FURTHER
- **118** Breathe into being
- **122** Morning meditation
- **126** Embrace the day

130 Meet the experts

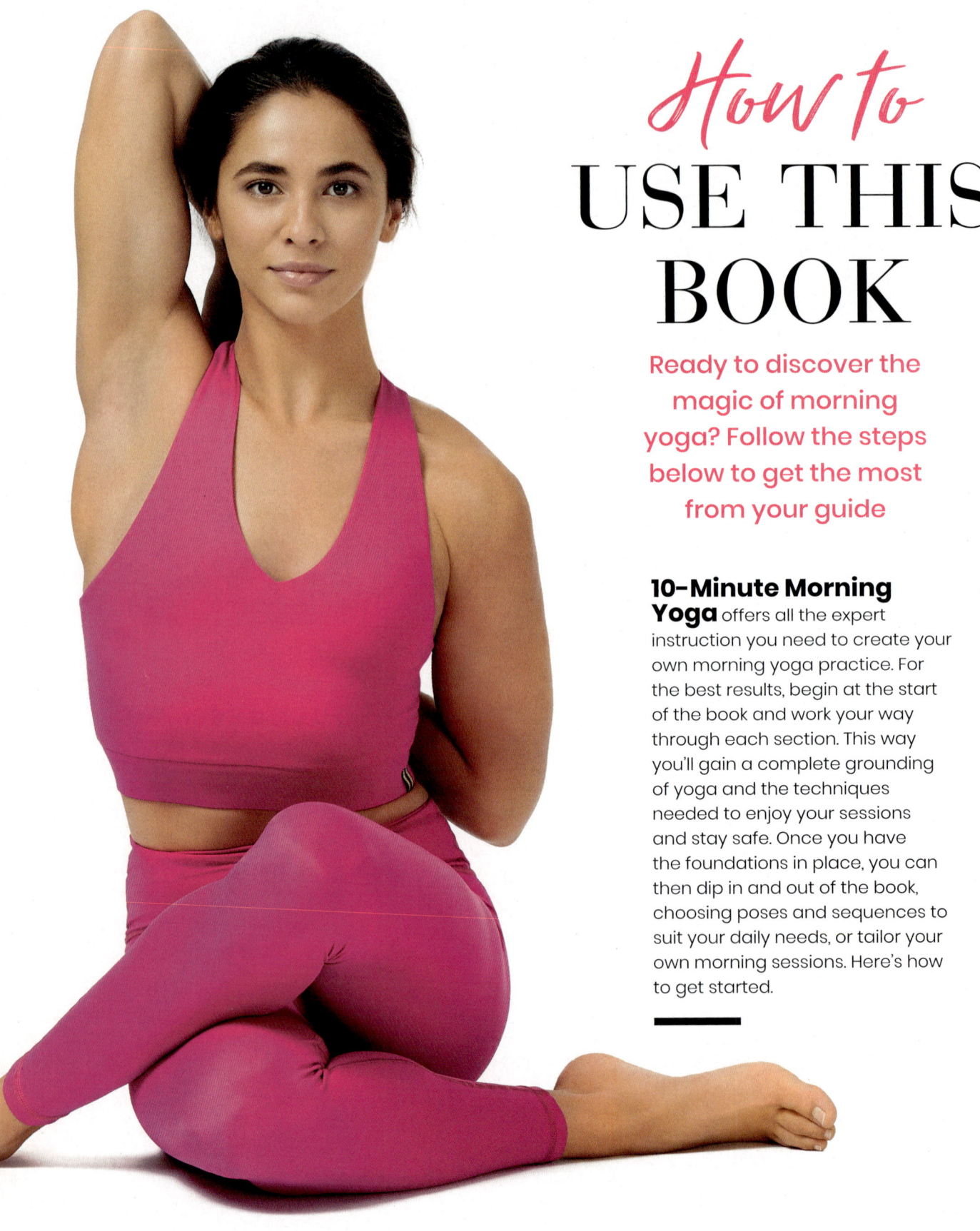

How to USE THIS BOOK

Ready to discover the magic of morning yoga? Follow the steps below to get the most from your guide

10-Minute Morning Yoga offers all the expert instruction you need to create your own morning yoga practice. For the best results, begin at the start of the book and work your way through each section. This way you'll gain a complete grounding of yoga and the techniques needed to enjoy your sessions and stay safe. Once you have the foundations in place, you can then dip in and out of the book, choosing poses and sequences to suit your daily needs, or tailor your own morning sessions. Here's how to get started.

Before you start

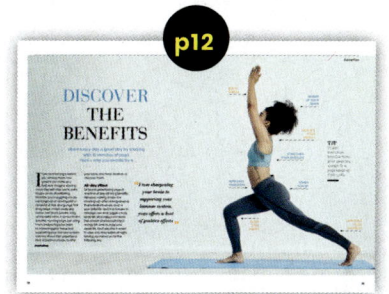

1 Discover the benefits
We reveal the amazing mind and body benefits of practising morning yoga. Discover how it can help you ease stiff muscles, kickstart your metabolism and sharpen your focus, then discover some of the best poses for every goal.

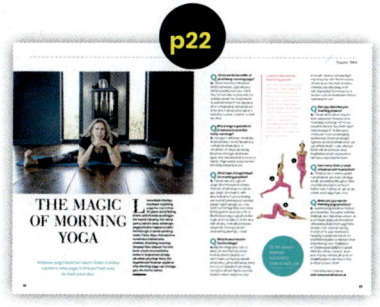

2 Meet your instructor
Top yoga teacher Laura Gate-Eastley explains why yoga is the perfect way to start your day and offers her tips and favourite poses for morning practice.

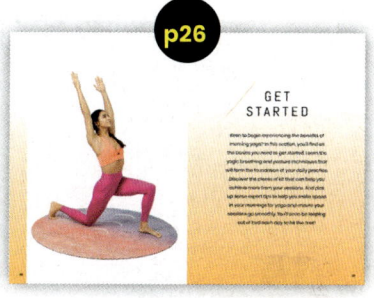

3 Get started
Understanding the foundations of yoga will ensure you enjoy your daily practice to the full. In this section, you'll discover the breathing and posture techniques you need, plus handy yoga props and kit.

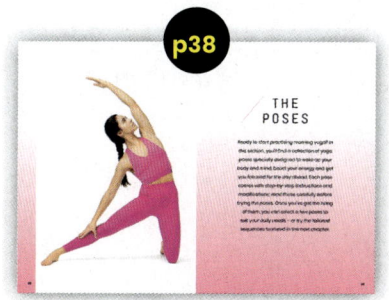

4 Learn the poses
Now it's time to try the yoga poses that will form the basis of your sessions. Each pose comes with step-by-step instructions; read these first to avoid injury or strain. You'll also learn the benefits each pose offers so you can tailor your practice to your needs.

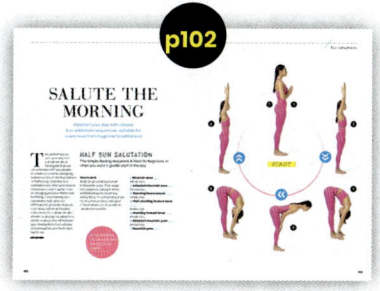

5 Try the sequences
Once you're familiar with the poses, you can combine them into flowing yoga sequences. In this section, you'll find energising Sun salutations plus four therapeutic sequences for daily life created by teacher Laura Gate-Eastley.

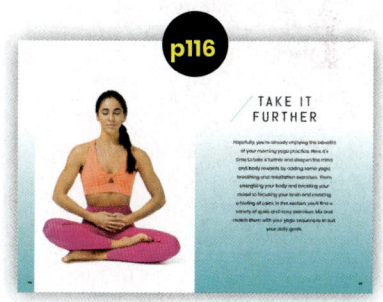

6 Deepen your practice
Breathwork and meditation exercises are also a key part of yoga. In this section, meditation teacher Ali Roff Farrar and breathwork expert Hanna-Jade Browne offer easy exercises to enhance your sessions.

MORNING MIRACLE

Sunrise yoga is an ancient tradition that will transform your life for the better

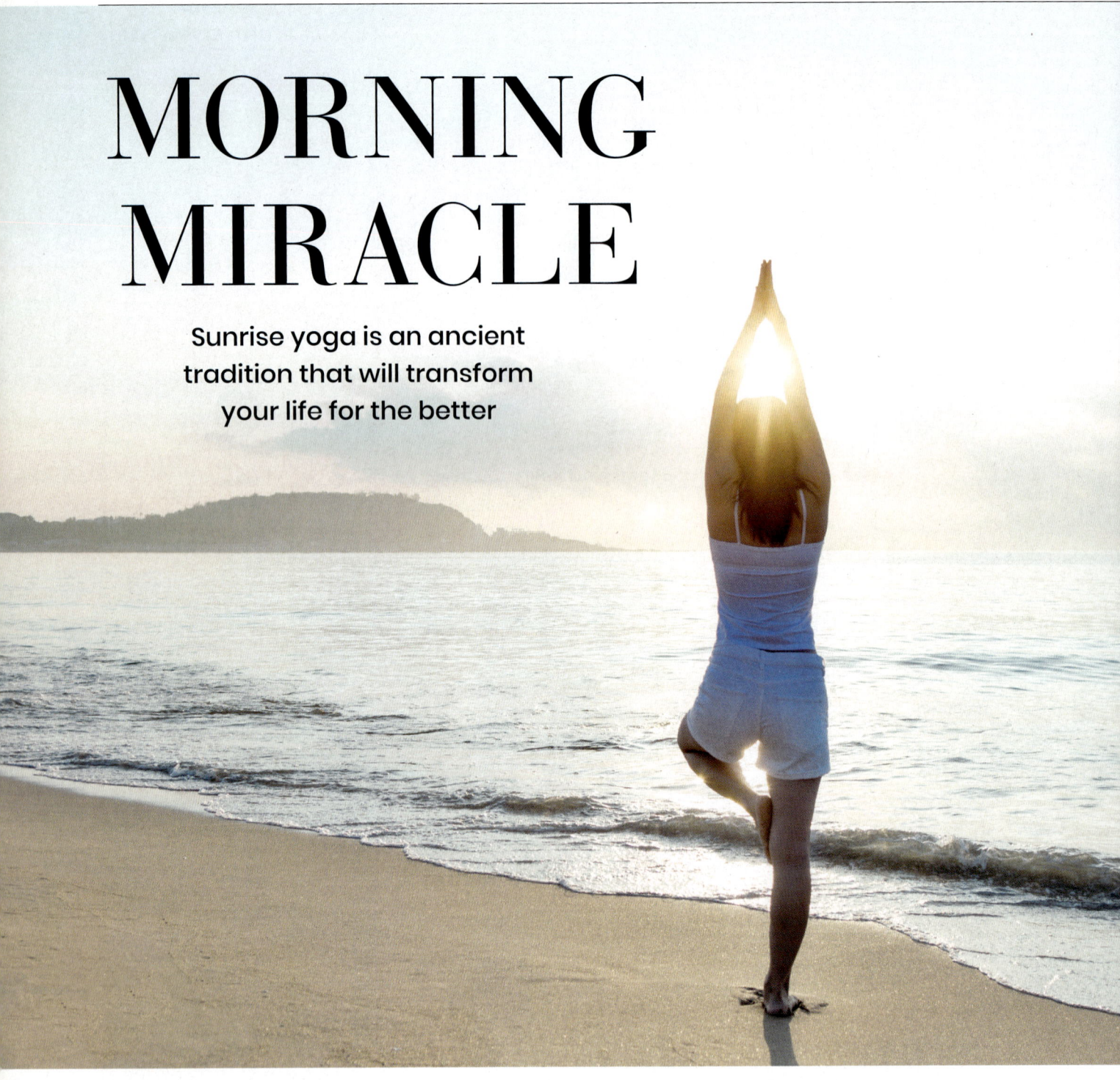

Picture the scene: it's morning and the first rays of sunlight are shining through your bedroom window. You wake up gently, feeling happy, refreshed and ready to embrace the day. Your body feels supple and energised, your mind calm and alert and the face that greets you in the bathroom mirror is glowing and radiant. With plenty of time on your hands before your working day begins, you do a short session of yoga, then shower and enjoy a healthy breakfast while catching up on the morning's news.

Doesn't sound like your average morning? Don't worry, you're not alone. Unless you're an early bird, mornings can be a stressful time of day, as you scramble out of bed and rush to get ready for work or organise the family. Sometimes, the day feels exhausting before it's even begun!

Yoga SOS

The idea of adding yoga into your busy morning may seem unrealistic. You're probably wondering how you'd find the time – after all, yoga is often associated with rest and relaxation. But think again! Traditionally, yoga is practised at sunrise because this is when the mind is most still and there are least distractions. Furthermore, far from just being relaxing, yoga

Introduction

The five principles of yoga

- **Exercise** In yoga, exercise comes in the form of the poses or 'asanas' which stretch, tone and strengthen your body.
- **Breathing** Connecting to your breath during yoga helps deepen your practice. Breathwork or Pranayama is used to achieve specific goals, from calming your mind to energising your body.
- **Relaxation** Yoga philosophy recognises that regular rest and relaxation —during practice and in daily life — releases tension and recharges your body.
- **Meditation** A key part of yoga, meditation helps you control and focus your mind. Even a few minutes a day can help.
- **Diet** Yogis recommend a simple, natural and ideally vegetarian diet to promote good health. You should eat mindfully, until you are 80 per cent full.

> YOGA WAKES UP YOUR BODY AND MIND, EASING STIFF LIMBS AND JOINTS.

offers a multitude of physical and mental benefits that can transform your daily life for the better, especially when practised first thing. And while a long session of yoga is lovely when you have the time, all you need to reap the rewards and turn your day around is 10 minutes!

Traditional practice

Meaning 'to yoke' or 'to unite', yoga connects your mind, body and spirit and brings you into harmony with your environment, helping you feel more at home in your body and in the outside world. In The Yoga Sutras, written around 2,000 years ago, Indian sage Patanjali described yoga as a practice for 'calming the fluctuations of the mind'. The physical yoga practice we're familiar with today was originally used to prepare the body for meditation to help further achieve these goals.

Yoga was introduced to the West by BKS Iyengar – the founder of Iyengar yoga – and has since branched into many styles of physical practice, from dynamic Ashtanga yoga to relaxing Yin yoga. Despite their differences, all forms of yoga have a similar aim – to stretch and strengthen your body and bring you into a state of inner calm and wellbeing. At its most basic, yoga helps you connect your mind and body through movement, mindfulness and breath to create optimum wellbeing.

Transform your day

In this sense, yoga is the perfect antidote to 21st century living, offering you much-needed space to breathe, move and look inwards. Practised first thing in the morning, yoga gently wakes up your body and mind, easing stiff limbs and joints, kickstarting your metabolism and priming your brain for the day ahead. Make time to spend just 10 minutes practising the poses and sequences in 10-Minute Morning Yoga and you'll soon find your energy levels improve. Your body will feel fitter and stronger and you'll start the day feeling calm and alert. You'll sleep better at night, find it easier to get up in the morning and discover you have more time on your hands than ever. Before long, you'll wonder how you managed without sunrise yoga!

DISCOVER THE BENEFITS

Make every day a good day by starting with 10 minutes of yoga. Here's why you should try it

If you've tried yoga before, you already know how great it can make you feel. Now imagine starting every day with that same calm, happy sense of wellbeing. Whether you're juggling a busy work agenda or dealing with a houseful of kids, doing yoga first thing helps makes every day better. And that's just the icing on the cake when it comes to the benefits morning yoga can bring. From sharpening your brain to improving your focus and supporting your immune system, science shows that yoga has a host of positive effects to offer your body and mind. Read on to discover more.

All-day effect
Of course, practising yoga at any time of day will bring benefits. However, making time in the morning can offer striking rewards that extend into every area of your daily life. You'll find it easier to manage your time, juggle a busy to-do list, stay happy and stress free at work and have plenty of energy left over to enjoy your social life. You'll also find it easier to relax and sleep better at night, leaving you refreshed for the following day.

> *"From sharpening your brain to supporting your immune system, yoga offers a host of positive effects"*

Benefits

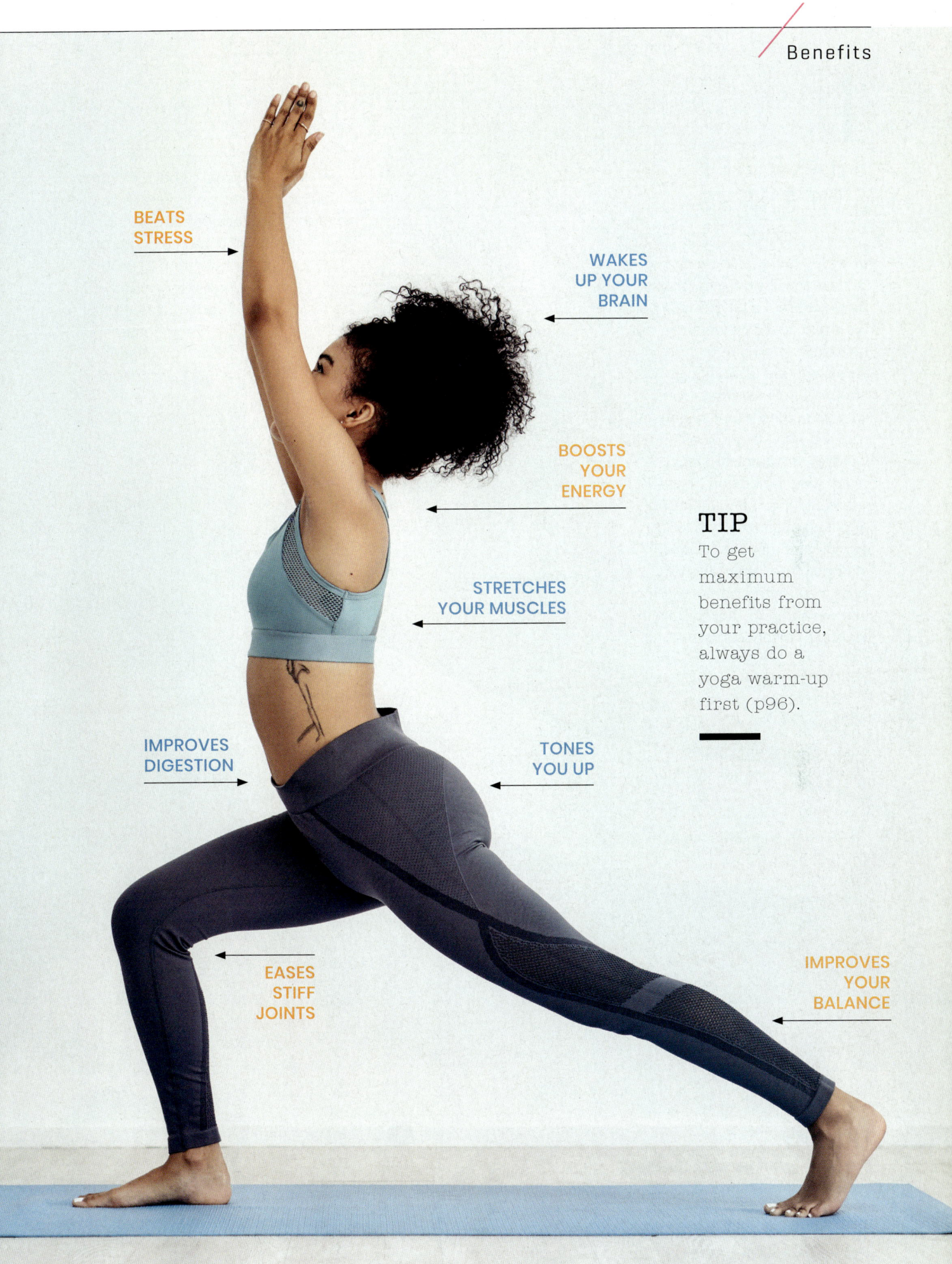

BEATS STRESS

WAKES UP YOUR BRAIN

BOOSTS YOUR ENERGY

STRETCHES YOUR MUSCLES

IMPROVES DIGESTION

TONES YOU UP

EASES STIFF JOINTS

IMPROVES YOUR BALANCE

TIP
To get maximum benefits from your practice, always do a yoga warm-up first (p96).

1
SHAKE OFF STIFFNESS

Hands up who feels a bit stiff and achy first thing in the morning? Don't worry, it's normal for our bodies to feel a bit creaky when we wake up. While we sleep, our muscles stiffen due to inactivity. That's why we get the urge to stretch when we wake – and why it's so important to get moving first thing. But, as we age or suffer from injury, aches and pains can become more common and disabling. Ageing causes the cartilage in our joints to dry out causing stiffness, and inflammation processes in the body 'switch on' in the morning, causing pain in injured or arthritic joints.

Morning yoga gently activates your muscles and joints to help you feel less creaky and more supple. By moving your joints through their full range of motion, yoga transports water and nutrients into your joints, spinal discs and cartilage,

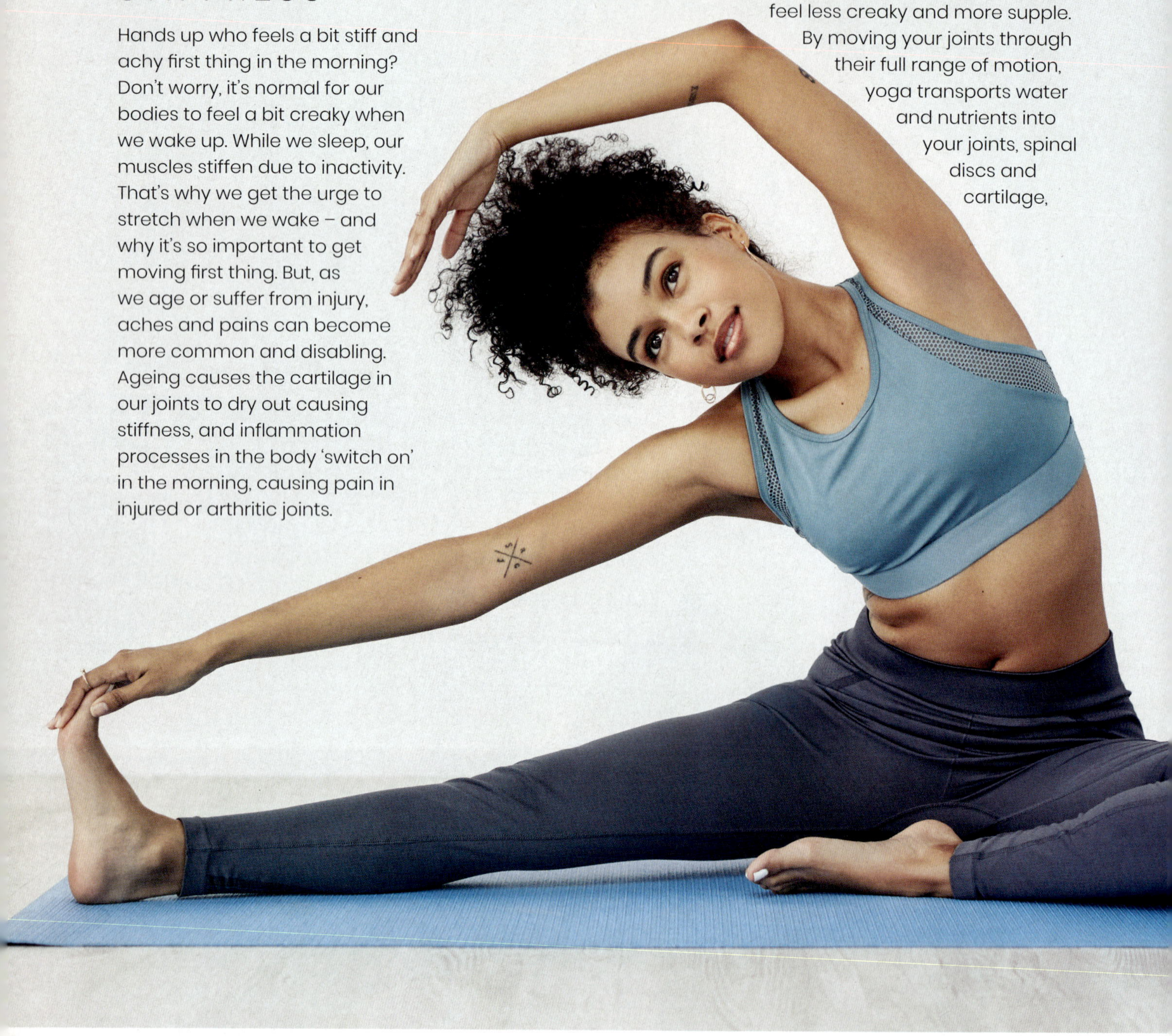

TRY THIS
Cat/Cow (p80) gently activates your body (1). Spine roll (p101) wakes up your body (2), while Tiger flow (p99) stretches your shoulders and thighs (3).

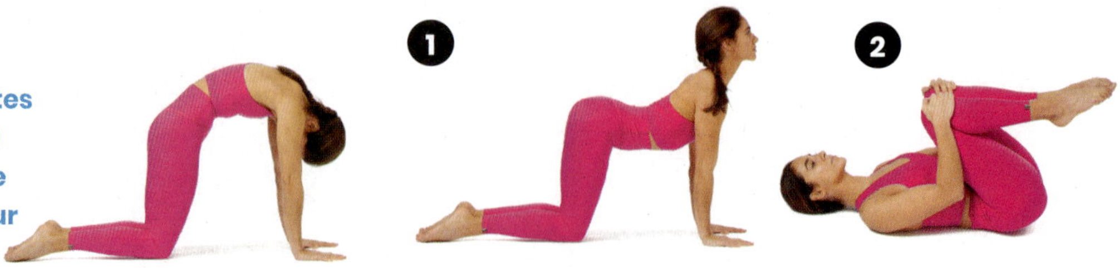

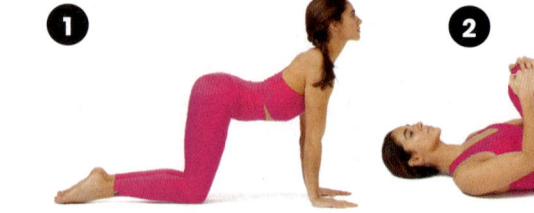

Benefits

TIP
Starting your day feeling supple will help reduce the strain of sitting at a desk.

---

keeping them lubricated and healthy. It also lengthens the connective tissue, muscles and ligaments between your joints, allowing you to become flexible again.

Plenty of studies show that yoga can improve back and joint pain and reduce the need for medication. One Indian study of people taking medication for rheumatoid arthritis found that, after eight weeks of yoga, markers of inflammation in their blood fell significantly, compared with people who didn't practise yoga. Active people are less likely to experience morning stiffness than inactive people and yoga is the perfect choice to start your day.

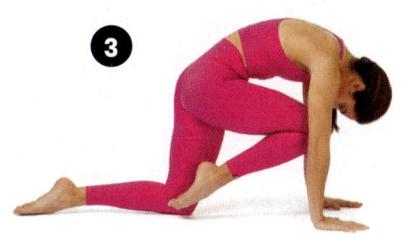

2 ENERGISE YOUR BODY

Yoga may be known for its calming, soothing benefits but it can also be stimulating and energising. Even if you feel tired when you wake up in the morning, a short yoga session is guaranteed to leave you feeling awake and alive. A study at the University of Waterloo in Canada, found that Hatha yoga effectively improves energy levels. Scientists believe this is because it improves your circulation, stimulates your brain, releases muscle tension and triggers the release of feel-good endorphins.

Unlike other forms of exercise that can leave you feeling exhausted, yoga incorporates periods of rest that keep your body refreshed and energised. For instance, you might rest in Child's pose (p86) or Forward bend (p42) in between challenging poses or relax in Corpse pose (p92) at the end of a sequence. Backbend poses are proven to be particularly good for energising and refreshing your mind and body. They extend your spine and open up your chest, allowing you to breathe more fully and oxygenate your lungs, energising your body. Sun salutation sequences (p102) are also designed to build your energy and are perfect for morning practice.

TRY THIS
Practise energising backbend poses such as Locust (p76) (1) or Cobra (p72) (2), or revitalising Bhastrika breath (p120) (3).

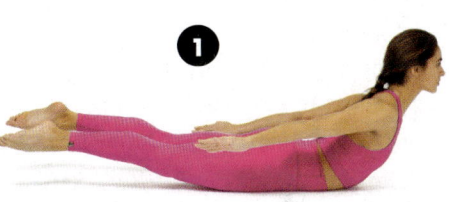

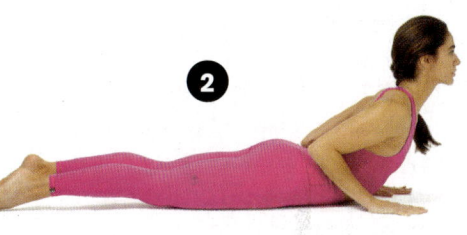

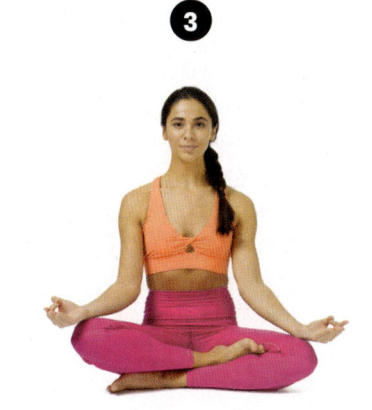

TIP
Woken up feeling exhausted? Try the Energise your day sequence (p108).

3
KEEP YOUR CALM

Are your mornings a frenzied blur as you rush to get ready for work while making breakfast for the family or walking the dog? Setting your alarm a little earlier each day and making space for 10 minutes of yoga first thing will settle your nervous system and allow you to start the day feeling calm and collected. Levels of stress hormones in the body are naturally high in the mornings (to help us wake up). Add everyday stress into the equation and the hormone levels soar higher, putting your body in 'fight or flight' mode and leaving you feeling anxious and jangly. Not a great way to start your working day! Doing yoga triggers the body's parasympathetic nervous system which slows your heart rate, lowers blood pressure and stimulates digestion, giving you a sense of relaxed wellbeing. One study on a group of people with depression, published in the Indian Journal of Psychiatry, found that levels of the stress hormone, cortisol, dropped significantly after they did three months of yoga. The researchers concluded that yoga works on the hypothalamus – the area of the brain associated with hormone release. That's why one of the easiest ways to calm down when you're stressed is to take slow, deep breaths. Add meditation to your sessions and the calming benefits magnify, ensuring you don't get caught up in a cycle of negative thoughts and behaviour. You'll begin the day feeling clear headed, centred and able to make decisions more easily.

TIP
Improve your focus further by trying a morning meditation (p122).

TRY THIS
Good poses for soothing stress include Child's pose (p86) (1), Corpse pose (p92) (2) and Forward bend (p42) (3).

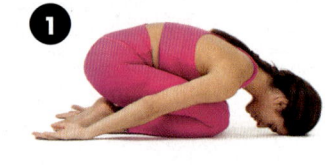

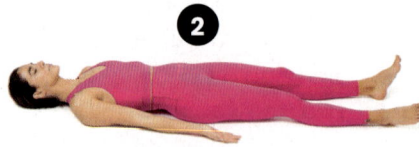

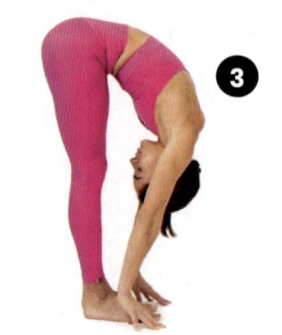

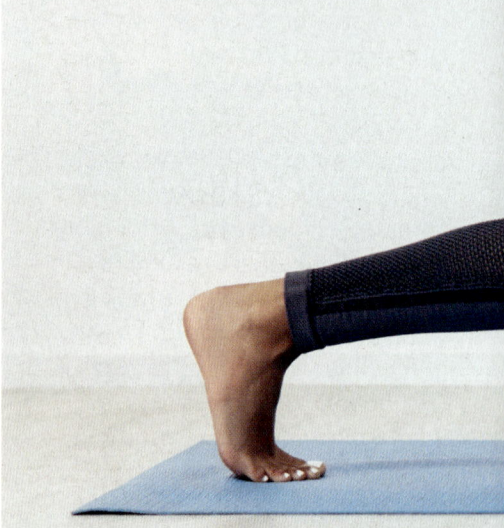

4
IMPROVE YOUR FOCUS

If your mind is always in a whirl first thing in the morning, doing yoga can help you clear your mind and prioritise things more efficiently. Focusing your brainpower on a set number of tasks, such as breathing and posture, reduces the processing of non-essential information, say scientists. Simply tuning into your breath and concentrating on

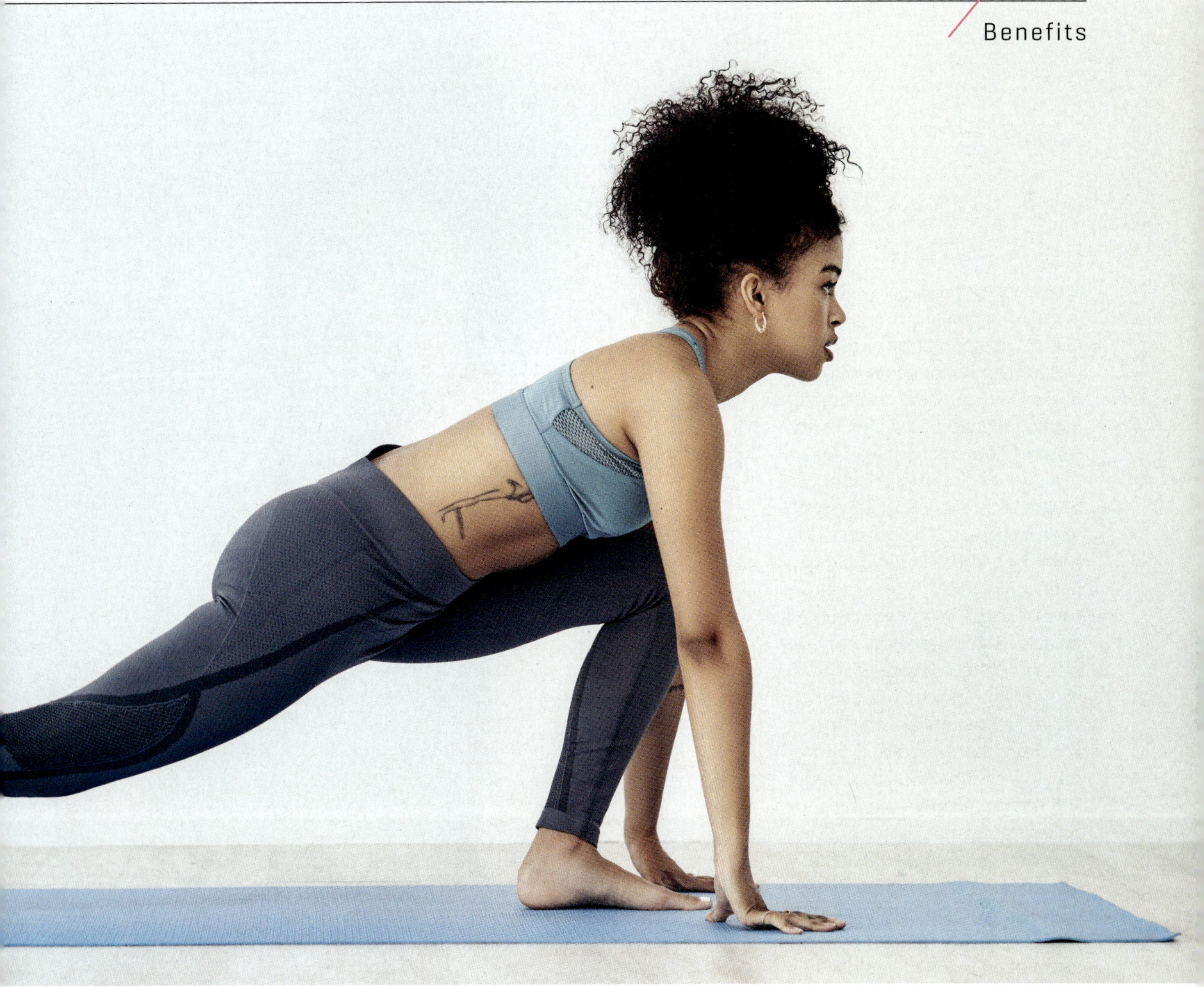

Benefits

performing poses and sequences helps rid your mind of distractions and anxiety. One study at the University of Waterloo in Canada found that just 10 minutes of mindful yoga significantly improved people's focus.
In the longer term, scientists believe that yoga affects the neural patterns of the brain in a positive way, improving your ability to concentrate. Balance poses are thought to be particularly effective for improving focus. As you concentrate on standing on one leg or balancing on your hands, you're forced to maintain your attention and this prepares your brain to deal effectively with whatever the day throws at you. Once you've mastered your balance, you'll find relaxing in these poses also has an empowering effect, giving you a sense of grounded confidence.

TRY THIS
One-legged balance poses such as Tree pose (p46) (1), Eagle (p56) (2) and Dancer pose (p58) (3) are particularly effective for improving focus.

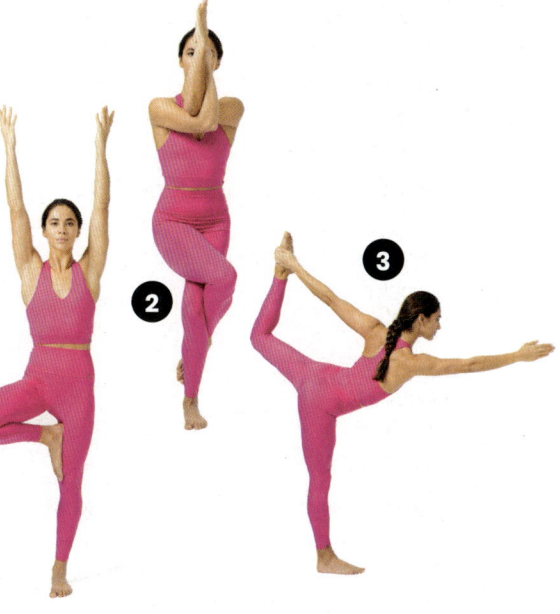

17

5
LIFT YOUR MOOD

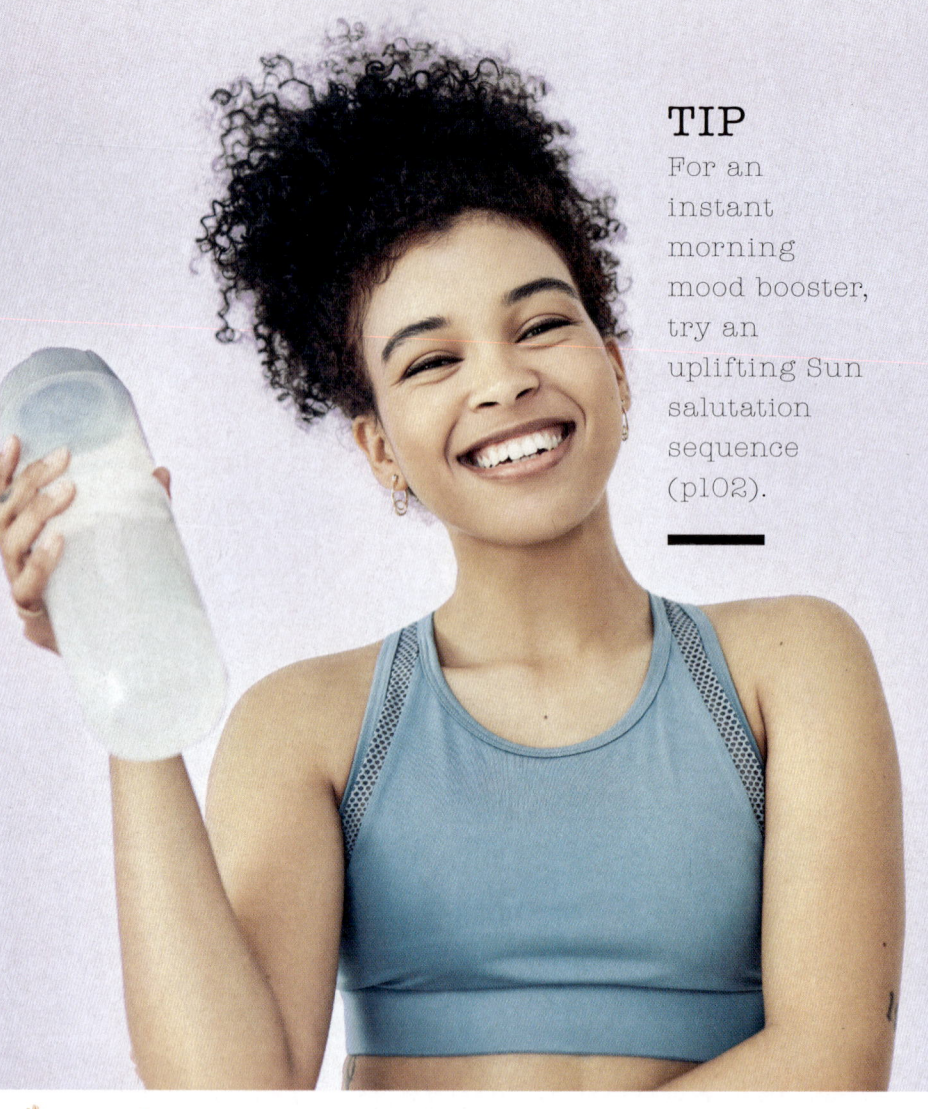

TIP
For an instant morning mood booster, try an uplifting Sun salutation sequence (p102).

Are you a bit grumpy first thing in the morning? You're not alone! Disrupted sleep, a long to-do list or simply not being 'a morning person' – there are many reasons our mood can be low first thing. Getting active is a proven way to lift your spirits but yoga could be just about the best exercise option there is. A research study, published in The Journal of Alternative and Complementary Medicine, followed two groups of people in a similar state of health. One group did a walking session three times a week, the other did yoga three times a week. After 12 weeks, the yoga group saw greater improvements in mood. The reason? The researchers believe yoga stimulates the brain to produce increased levels of an amino acid called gamma-aminobutyric acid (GABA B) which helps promote feelings of calm. GABA B activity tends to be lower in people with poor mood and anxiety.

Yoga can also improve your body confidence and self esteem due to its empowering postures. Simply standing or sitting up straight rather than slumping sends positive messages to your brain, improving your sense of wellbeing and happiness.

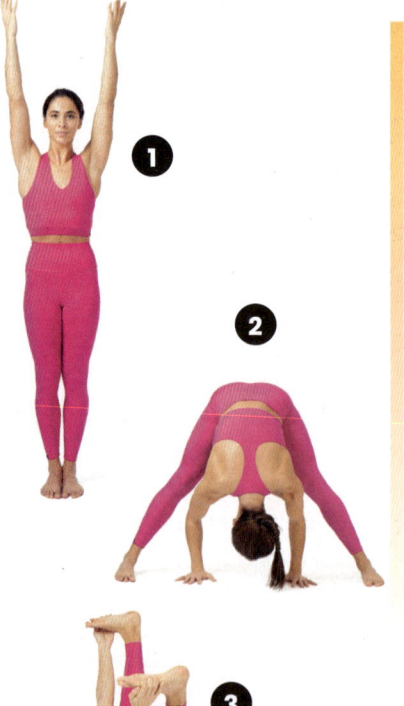

TRY THIS
Feel-good poses include Extended mountain pose (p41) (1), Wide-legged forward bend (p54) (2) and Happy baby (p101) (3).

How yoga beats stress

■ Your body's nervous system has two main branches — the sympathetic and parasympathetic systems. When you're under stress, the sympathetic nervous system is activated to prepare your body for 'fight or flight'. It releases the stress hormones adrenaline and cortisol, increases your heart rate and raises blood pressure. The parasympathetic system, sometimes called the 'rest and digest' system, has the opposite role, reducing stress hormone levels, lowering your blood pressure and heartbeat and preparing your body for rest. By deepening your breath and soothing your brain, yoga tells your body you're safe, triggering the parasympathetic system and allowing your body to settle into a calm state.

Benefits

6
RELEASE MUSCLE TENSION

Do you get backache from sitting at a desk all day or suffer headaches from staring at a computer screen? Daily life causes a build up of muscle tension that, left unaddressed, can take a toll on your health or lead to injury. Repetitive patterns of movement, sport or stress can cause your muscles to contract around the joints, limiting your range of movement and causing pain. Tension in one area of the body can lead to problems in another – even a tense, clenched jaw can affect your whole body. And, as the mind and body are linked, holding tension in your body can also cause fatigue and low mood.

As with any stretch-based exercise, yoga can help ease out tension from your muscles but, by incorporating the mindful breath, yoga can achieve greater results. By directing your breath towards areas of tension during a yoga pose, you can consciously help your muscles to relax and open your joints to allow energy to flow freely again. Yoga works on both sides of your body equally, gradually bringing it back into balance. It also helps erase unconscious postural habits, such as tensing areas of your body when you're under pressure. If you practise yoga in the mornings, you'll soon notice your posture starts to improve and your muscles will feel more relaxed.

TRY THIS

Ease tight hamstrings with Half-splits pose (p50) (1), release neck tension with Head rolls (p97) (2) and open your chest with Sphinx pose (p73) (3).

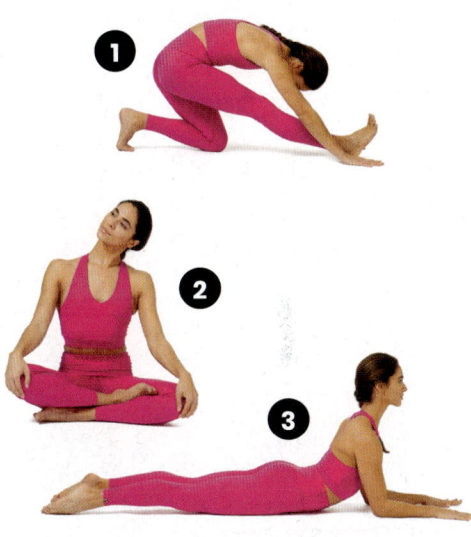

7
BOOST YOUR BRAIN

If you need to get your brain into gear in the morning, yoga is the answer. Studies show that just a short session of poses and sequences can stimulate brain function afterwards. One study at the University of Illinois, USA, found that a single yoga session improved participants' speed and accuracy when working on memory tests (a measure of the brain's ability to cope with new information). The effects were greater than for those doing aerobic exercise.

Like any exercise, yoga helps boost circulation, improving blood flow to the brain. But certain poses offer extra benefits.

Ever noticed that yogis are often depicted in Headstands and Shoulderstands? These inversion poses, where your head is lower than your legs, draw the blood supply to your brain, nourishing it with the oxygen and nutrients it needs to function well. You don't have to do a Headstand to reap the benefits.

As you'll find in this book, there are inversion poses for all levels of ability. They're perfect for when you need to refresh your brain, and also provide a break for tired legs. The mindful nature of yoga can also rejuvenate your brain, helping it re-focus its energies. For deeper benefits, try meditation (p122) – it's proven to increase creativity.

TRY THIS

For an instant brain boost, try inversion poses such as Bridge pose (p99) (1) and Downward-facing dog (p62) (2) or uplifting Upward-facing dog (p74) (3).

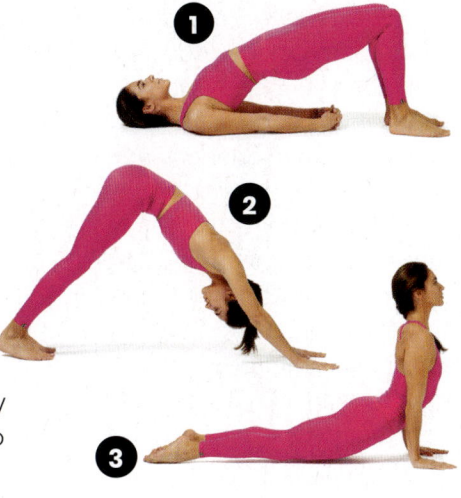

19

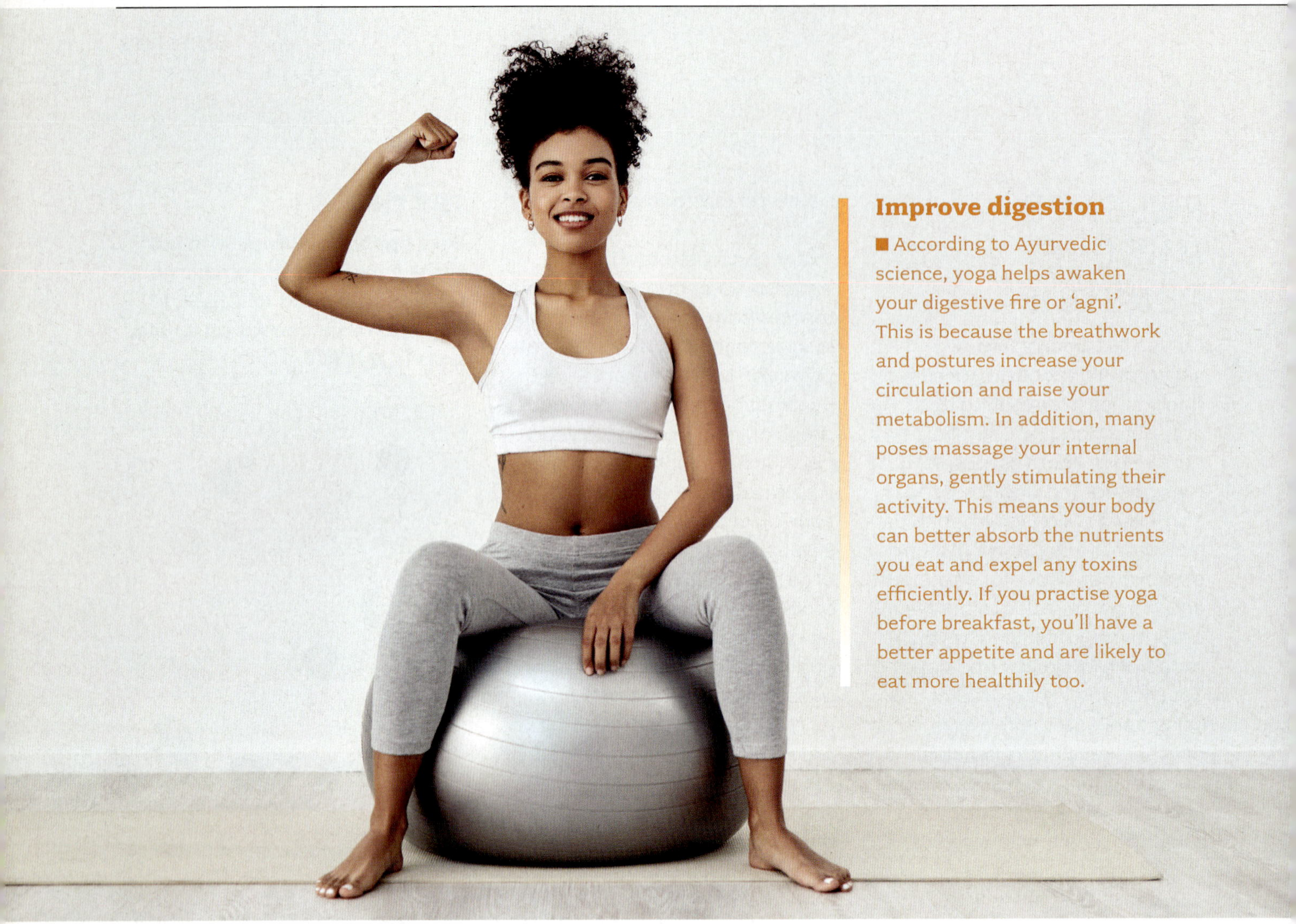

Improve digestion

■ According to Ayurvedic science, yoga helps awaken your digestive fire or 'agni'. This is because the breathwork and postures increase your circulation and raise your metabolism. In addition, many poses massage your internal organs, gently stimulating their activity. This means your body can better absorb the nutrients you eat and expel any toxins efficiently. If you practise yoga before breakfast, you'll have a better appetite and are likely to eat more healthily too.

8
GET IN SHAPE

Want to tone up or lose weight? You don't have to spend hours on the treadmill or sweating it out at the gym. By getting you moving and deepening your breathing, yoga boosts your metabolism, helping burn calories and stimulating your body's inner organs. If you choose more vigorous yoga sequences, you can burn more calories as you build up a sweat.

Research shows that practising yoga regularly can lead to lower body fat levels, a healthy body mass index (BMI), and a reduced waist-to-hip ratio. Studies also show that people who practise yoga have better appetite control, tend to eat more mindfully and maintain a healthy weight. By building lean muscle mass and stretching your muscles, yoga also improves your body tone, giving you a longer, leaner look. Meanwhile, improved posture helps you look slimmer and younger.

TRY THIS

Burn calories with Plank (p66) (1), improve your posture with Mountain pose (p40) (2) and tone your legs with Chair pose (p44) (3).

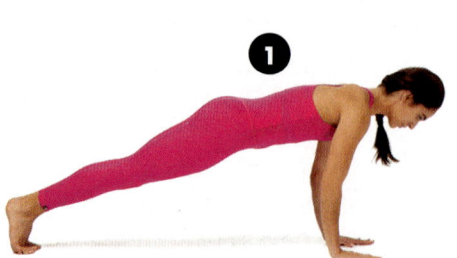
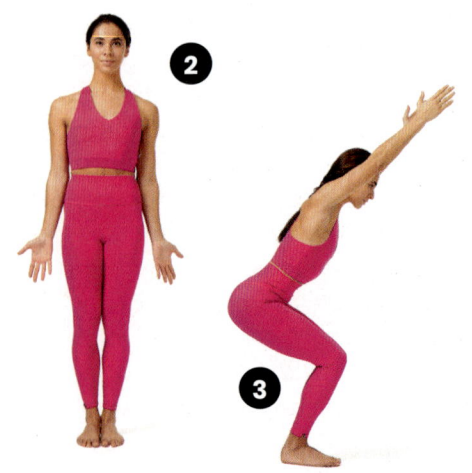

Benefits

9 SUPPORT YOUR IMMUNITY

Whether you want to optimise your wellbeing or stave off office germs, yoga can help keep you stay healthy by supporting your immune system. While vigorous exercise sometimes over-stresses the immune system, leaving you vulnerable to colds and infection, gentle exercise such as yoga helps stimulate the body's systems without strain. By boosting your circulation and lymphatic system, yoga enables your disease-fighting white blood cells to do their job properly. Science suggests yoga may reduce inflammation in the body that is linked to disease such as cancer.

Yoga also erases the stress that can compromise your immune system. Specific poses such as inversions are thought to be particularly good for boosting the lymphatic system. But the main thing is to create a regular, all-year-round yoga practice, even if it's just 10 minutes a day.

TRY THIS

To boost your lymphatic system, try Bridge pose (p99) (1). Stave off colds with Cobra (p72) (2) and strengthen your lungs with Easy pose (p31) (3).

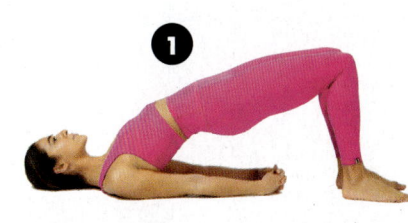

TIP
Inverted poses such as Bridge (p99) are said to help keep colds at bay.

10 LOOK AWAKE

Yoga doesn't just help you feel good, it makes you look good too. It's no coincidence that many yoga instructors look so youthful! By improving your posture, relaxing your facial muscles and boosting the supply of oxygen and nutrients to your skin, yoga helps you look years younger than your age. And the good news is, it can also give you an instant beauty boost in the morning, reviving tired-looking skin and giving you a radiant glow and sparkling eyes.

Certain yoga poses are particularly known for their beauty benefits. Inversion poses and forward bends deliver fresh blood to your face, oxygenating and nourishing your skin, leaving your complexion bright. Twisting poses boost your lymphatic system and improve your digestion, helping your vital organs expel the toxins that can cause dull, sluggish skin. And backbend poses help open your chest to deepen your breathing and oxygenate your body. These poses also have the bonus of stretching your neck and lifting and firming your jaw line. If you've ever noticed how refreshed you look after a yoga class, this is why!

TRY THIS

To release tension in your face, try Lion's breath pose (p100) (1), aid detoxification with Easy twist (p96) (2) and tone your jawline with Camel pose (p78) (3).

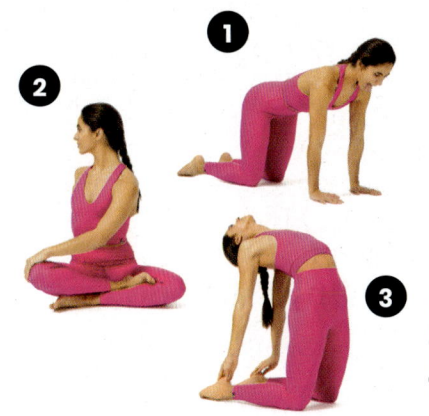

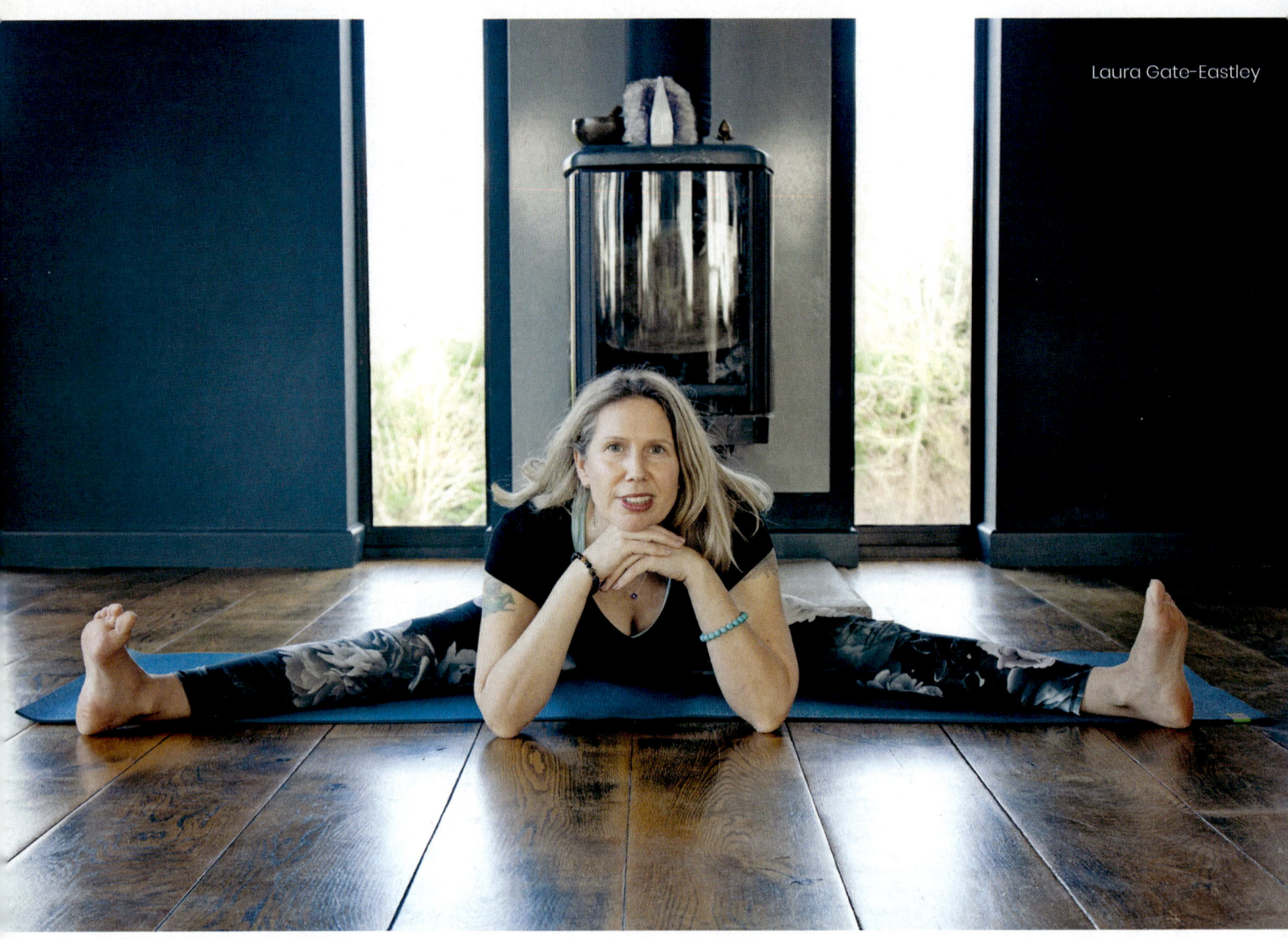

Laura Gate-Eastley

THE MAGIC OF MORNING YOGA

Vinyasa yoga teacher Laura Gate-Eastley explains why yoga is the perfect way to start your day

Laura Gate-Eastley has been teaching yoga for more than 20 years since falling in love with it while working in the music industry. For many years, Laura's daily Ashtanga yoga practice helped sustain her through a hectic working week. These days, she teaches numerous classes and retreats, including morning Vinyasa Flow classes. For this book, Laura has created a series of sequences to help you start your day. Here, the experienced teacher explains why morning yoga can change your life for the better.

Expert Q&A

Q What are the benefits of practising morning yoga?
A. 'I think morning is the best time to practise yoga as your body is rested and your mind has not yet been pulled into the outside world. You may intend to practise later in the day and then unexpected obstacles can arise and change your plans. A morning routine is easier to stick to, I find.'

Q Why is yoga a good form of exercise to practise in the mornings?
A. 'As yoga is a holistic modality that includes mindful breathing and some meditation or relaxation, it helps your body become stronger and more open, but also develop a sense of clarity. Yoga eases away tension, mentally and physically.'

Q What type of yoga is best for morning practice?
A. 'I would say any type of yoga. Sit or lie down for a few minutes of self enquiry before you begin, to check in with your baseline. If you're feeling exhausted (perhaps you've had a bad night's sleep), you may want something slow and close to the ground such as a Yin or Restorative yoga sequence. But if you want to ease in to the day with vitality, a mindful Vinyasa sequence can be just the exhilarating start you need.'

Q What is your ritual in the mornings?
A. 'My mornings start with a glass of warm lemon water. I move around quietly, so I don't wake up my household, otherwise I get pulled away from this much-needed time. I keep the lights off and light a candle instead which helps me stay in a calm space. I usually light my oil burner with frankincense oil and lie on the mat for a few minutes, just deciding what sort of practice to move into. It always ends in meditation: that is essential for me.'

Q Can you describe your morning classes?
A. 'I teach all levels of Vinyasa Flow classes on Tuesday and Thursday mornings. I think my students like the fact that I don't race through it. I build layers of deeper, more challenging options but there are always options, so nobody feels they are out of their depth. I also always finish with breathwork and meditation which my students tell me is important to them.'

Q How many times a week should we aim to practise?
A. 'Three times a week is great, but whatever you can manage works. Sometimes life gets in the way. Five minutes is so much better than nothing, so aim to do a little most days if you can.'

Q What are your tips for morning yoga practice?
A. 'Avoid eating breakfast before your practice. The poses will help wake up your digestive system, so you'll really enjoy your breakfast afterwards. Build in enough time to enjoy that without having to rush on to your next event. Keeping a notebook handy for any little snippets of wisdom that arise during your meditation or Corpse pose (p92) is a good idea, too. When you turn down your mental chatter, all sorts of insightful gems can rise to the surface of your mind!'

→ For more about Laura, visit, www.lauralotus.co.uk

Laura's favourite morning poses

'My three favourite morning poses are a High lunge (p52) (A) to stretch every part of my body (my hip flexors are always a little stiff and thank me for this); Puppy dog (p100) (B) which opens up my lungs and puts me in a good mood; and Eagle (p56) (C), especially if I am linking it into a pose such as a Warrior 3. I like the feeling of strength and grace it delivers.'

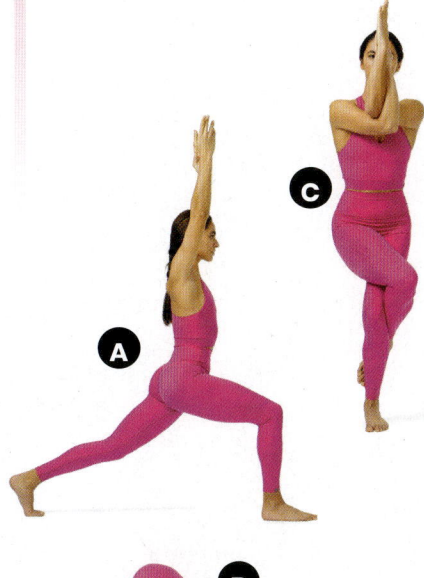

TO TRY LAURA'S MORNING SEQUENCES, TURN TO PAGE 108

HOW TO BE AN EARLY BIRD

Are you more owl than lark? Follow these easy steps and learn to love your mornings

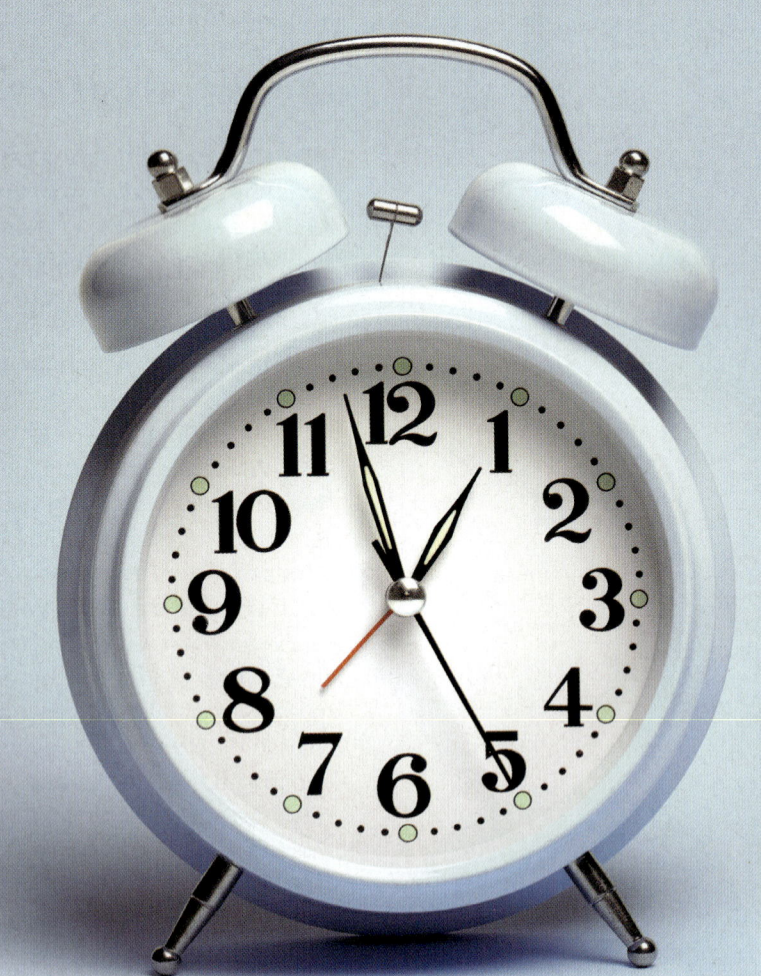

Do you struggle to get up in the morning? The good news is you can adjust your inner body clock to wake up earlier every day, feeling raring to go, just by making a few easy lifestyle changes.

Even if you're a natural night owl, you'll soon find you enjoy the peace and breathing space your early mornings bring and will head into the day feeling energised and ready to take on the world. And, as an early bird, research shows you're likely to be happier and more productive than night owls. So what are you waiting for? Start following these tips today and you'll soon start to see the benefits!

Morning tips

1 SWITCH OFF SCREENS
Do you spend your evenings watching TV or scrolling social media on your phone? The blue light from digital devices can disrupt your circadian rhythms, telling your body it's time to be awake and alert. It also reduces the production of the sleep hormone, melatonin, that helps you fall asleep. Try switching off your digital devices an hour before bed and wind down with some gentle yoga, a relaxing bath or good book. Keep digital gadgets out of the bedroom and turn down the lights in your living room and bedroom while you prepare for bed.

2 CHANGE YOUR BEDTIME
Your body clock is happiest when you stick to a regular bedtime. And if you want to wake up earlier in the morning, feeling full of beans, you'll need to hit the sack earlier too. To begin with, try to move your bedtime back by 15 minutes and gradually shift it earlier. Set bedtime reminders on your phone to help you make the habit. Don't worry if you struggle at the start – it takes a couple of weeks to create a new habit – but soon you'll start to feel sleepy earlier in the evenings.

3 EAT EARLIER
It's not just your bedtime that helps set your body clock – your meal times also play a role. Research shows that sticking to regular meal times is key. Aim to eat breakfast soon after you rise. This tells your brain and metabolism that it's time to wake up. Try to set regular times for your lunch and dinner too. And eat your evening meal before 8pm to allow plenty of time for your body to digest. This tells your brain it's time to rest.

4 LET THE LIGHT IN
As soon as you wake, open your bedroom blinds to let daylight in. Not only does the natural light help you feel alert, it also releases feel-good chemicals in the brain. Once you're up and about, try to get outside as soon as possible for at least 20 minutes. Research shows that exposure to the early morning light (whether it's sunny or not) helps regulate your body's sleep/wake cycle, ensuring you'll sleep soundly at night and wake up feeling refreshed. Breathing the fresh morning air will also energise your body.

5 REMOVE OBSTACLES
What is it you particularly dread about the prospect of an early morning? Try to identify any pitfalls that may get in the way of you rising early. For instance, if you're worried you'll feel tired, aim to go to bed earlier. If you think you won't be organised in time, prepare your clothes and work bag or gym kit the night before. If you always feel grumpy in the morning, try creating an uplifting morning playlist to boost your mood.

Shift your body clock
Research published in the journal Sleep Medicine confirms it's possible for a night owl to shift their body clock to become more of a 'morning person'. In a study by the UK Universities of Birmingham and Surrey, 22 night owls were asked to go to bed two to three hours before their usual bedtime and wake two to three hours before their regular waking up time for three weeks. They ate breakfast on waking and had dinner before 7pm. Results showed the volunteers were able to shift their waking time back by two hours without reducing sleep duration. They also saw improvements in their reaction time and reported feeling less depressed and stressed.

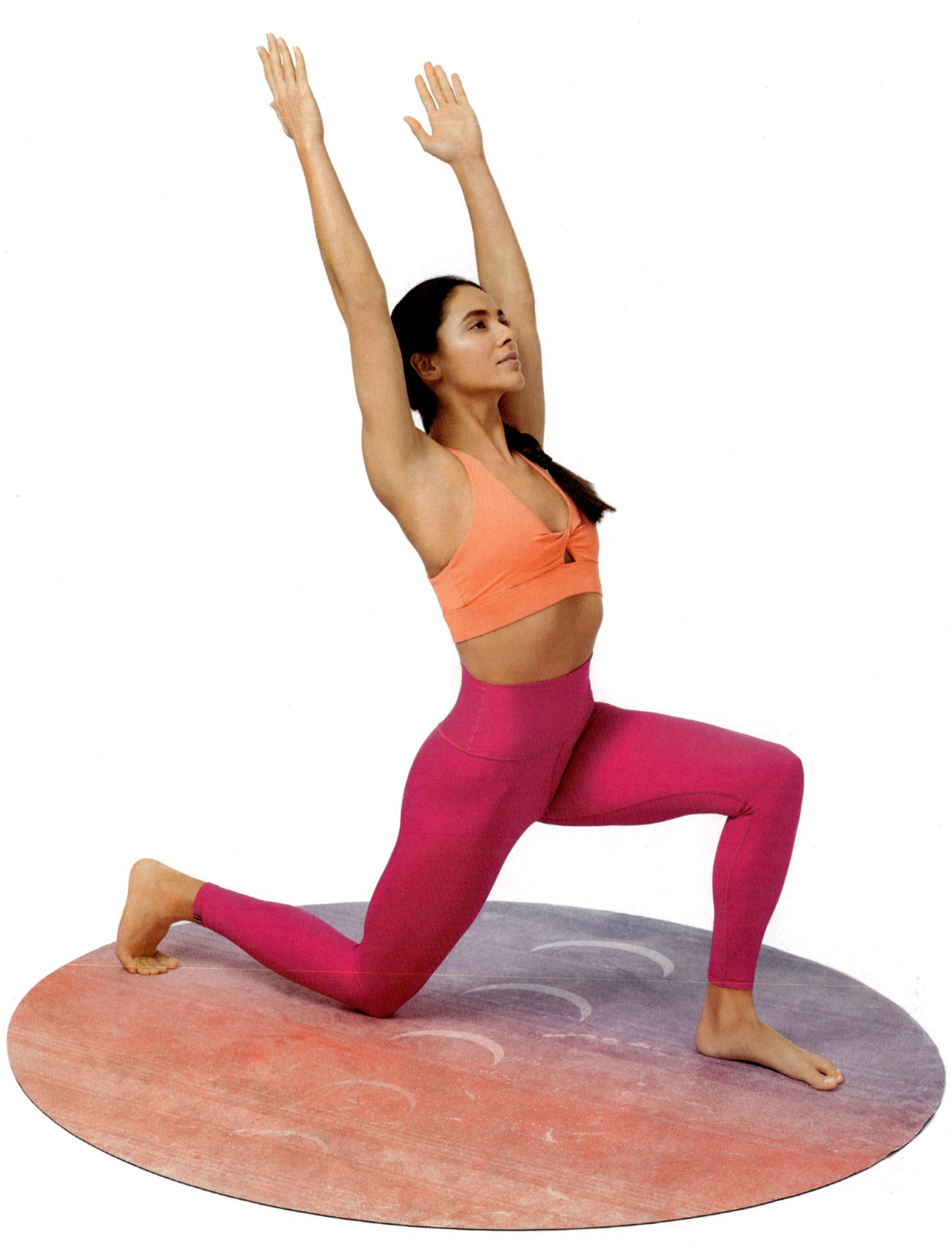

GET STARTED

Keen to begin experiencing the benefits of morning yoga? In this section, you'll find all the basics you need to get started. Learn the yogic breathing and posture techniques that will form the foundation of your daily practice. Discover the pieces of kit that can help you achieve more from your sessions. And pick up some expert tips to help you make space in your mornings for yoga and ensure your sessions go smoothly. You'll soon be leaping out of bed each day to hit the mat!

Breathing BASICS

Learning how to breathe well is the foundation of your yoga practice. It can also transform your daily life

From the minute you wake up in the morning, your breath carries you through the day. But, did you know the way you breathe can have a big impact on your health and happiness? The pressures of day-to-day life often lead to shallow breathing, depriving your body's cells of the oxygen and nutrients they need to function properly. This means your brain, muscles and vital organs don't perform as well as they should. Shallow breathing also triggers the release of stress hormones such as cortisol which, in the long-term, can lead to ill-health and burn out.

Breathe better

In yoga, breath control is key because it connects your mind and body and brings you into the moment. Yogic breathing also ensures your body is fully oxygenated, supporting your practice and bringing you back to optimum health. In addition, there are yogic breath-control exercises, known as Pranayama (p118), after 'Prana' which means energy and 'yama' which means to extend. By learning to direct your breath in specific ways you can cleanse, calm or energise your body and mind. But the starting point of yoga is to simply tune into your breath and learn to consciously control it. Here's how.

THE YOGIC BREATH

This is a key technique to learn for the basis of your yoga practice. It's often practised at the beginning of a yoga session to calm your breath and help you tune into your body before practising the postures.

1 Sit or lie in a comfortable position and, once you're settled, gently close your eyes.
2 Take a couple of deep breaths in through your nose and out through your mouth, releasing any tension as you exhale. Then let your breath settle and feel your mind start to calm down.
3 Tune into your breath and your natural breathing rhythm. Is it fast or slow, shallow or deep? Try counting the length of each in-breath and out-breath, noticing the slight pause in between.
4 Gently deepen your breath, breathing into your belly. Can you feel your diaphragm lifting and ribcage expanding as you inhale, and lowering as you exhale?
5 Now place one hand on your abdomen and the other on your chest. Breathe into your belly, then your ribs and finally all the way up to your chest. As you exhale, reverse the process, emptying your breath from your chest, then your ribs and finally your belly. To guide you, feel the rise and fall with your hands.
6 Continue for a few slow breaths, then gently let your breathing return to normal.

Breathing tips

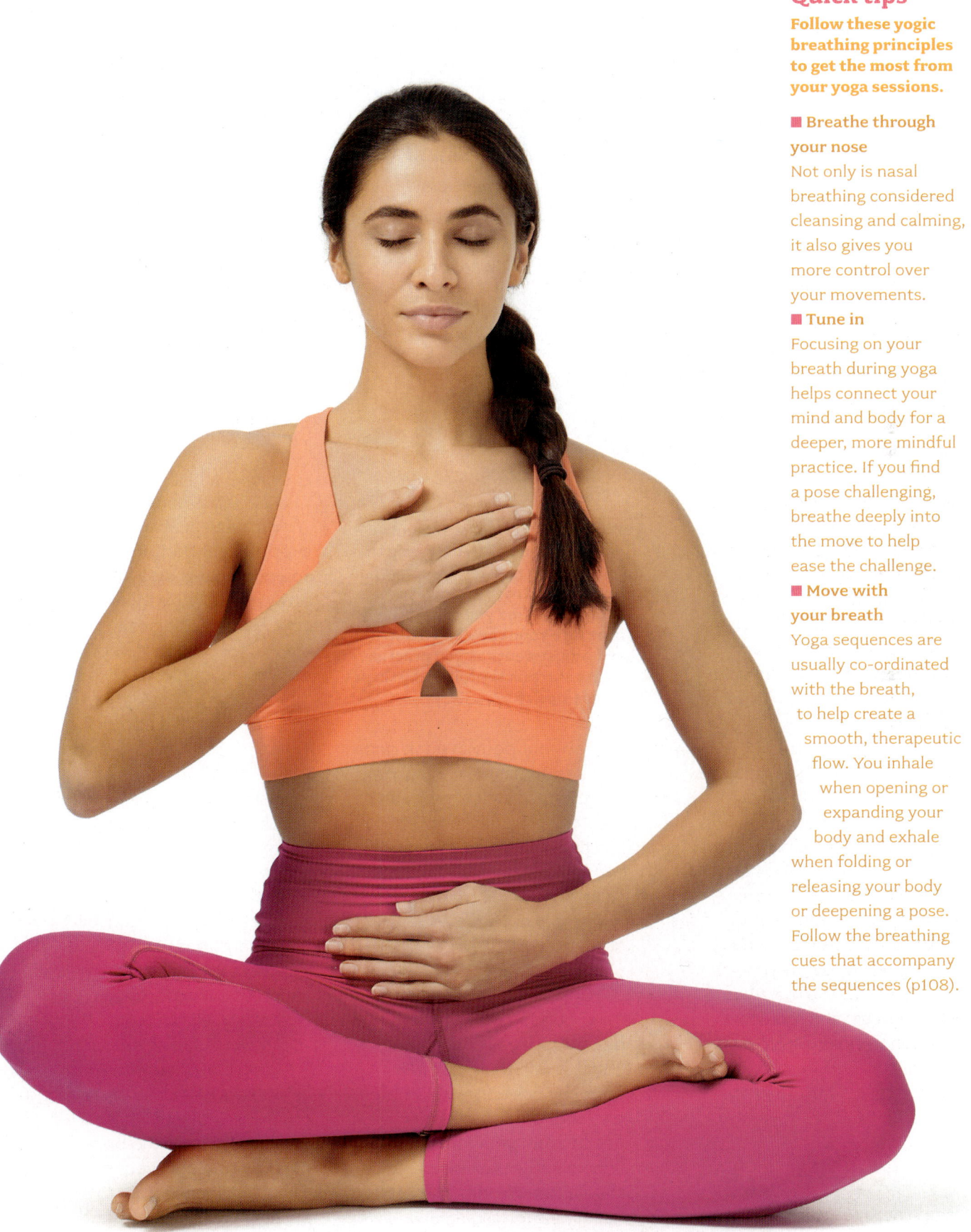

Quick tips

Follow these yogic breathing principles to get the most from your yoga sessions.

■ Breathe through your nose
Not only is nasal breathing considered cleansing and calming, it also gives you more control over your movements.

■ Tune in
Focusing on your breath during yoga helps connect your mind and body for a deeper, more mindful practice. If you find a pose challenging, breathe deeply into the move to help ease the challenge.

■ Move with your breath
Yoga sequences are usually co-ordinated with the breath, to help create a smooth, therapeutic flow. You inhale when opening or expanding your body and exhale when folding or releasing your body or deepening a pose. Follow the breathing cues that accompany the sequences (p108).

PERFECT POSTURE

Knowing the fundamentals of yoga alignment will help you practise safely

Whether you spend your days hunched over a laptop or standing on your feet, daily life can take a toll on your posture, causing back pain, headaches and muscle tension. Over the years, poor posture can cause you to look and feel older than your years. Practising yoga regularly helps redress the damage, stretching your body and strengthening your core to support your spine. By making you more self aware, yoga also helps you notice when you're slouching and encourages you to sit and stand tall. The more you practise yoga, the more this body awareness will grow.

Alignment tips

Yoga has its own posture and alignment guidelines. Putting these foundations in place deepens your practice and reduces injury risk. Soon, you'll find you instinctively tune into your body and make self-adjustments as you practise. To get started, try following these simple tips:

1 Scan your body in each pose to see how it feels. Tune into your breath and consciously relax any part of your body not involved in holding the pose. If you feel pain, stop and make adjustments using any props necessary or try again another day.

2 Check your body is firmly grounded by ensuring any parts of your body in contact with the mat are correctly positioned to create a strong foundation. You may need to root your feet into the floor or settle the sitting bones of your bottom into your mat, for instance.

3 Keep your core engaged to protect your back and support your body in the poses. You can do this by gently drawing your navel into your spine. It also helps strengthen and tone your abdominal muscles.

4 To stay stable and avoid strain during a pose, ensure your joints are always stacked – for instance knees over ankles or shoulders over wrists. In Mountain pose (p40), your knees should be aligned over your ankles and your pelvis over your knees. In Cat/Cow (p80), your shoulders should be stacked over your wrists and your hips over your knees.

5 To avoid straining your neck, keep it aligned with your spine. Read the pose instructions carefully and note whether you need to keep the back of your neck long, your chin tucked in and whether to gaze up, down or straight ahead.

/ The basics

How to sit

Many yoga warm-up and beginner poses are done from a sitting or kneeling position. Here's how to stay aligned.

STAFF POSE
Dandasana

This pose focuses your mind, stretches your back, opens your chest and shoulders and tones your arms and legs. It's harder to maintain than you think!

■ Sit on the floor with your legs together in front of you and your back straight.
■ Adjust the fleshy part of your bottom, rooting your sitting bones into the floor.
■ Press the backs of your thighs into the floor, then rotate your thighs slightly inwards.
■ Plant your hands beside your hips or on your lap, keep your shoulders down and relaxed. Look straight ahead and draw your chin in.
■ Flex your feet.
■ Inhale and lengthen your upper body.
■ Exhale and relax.

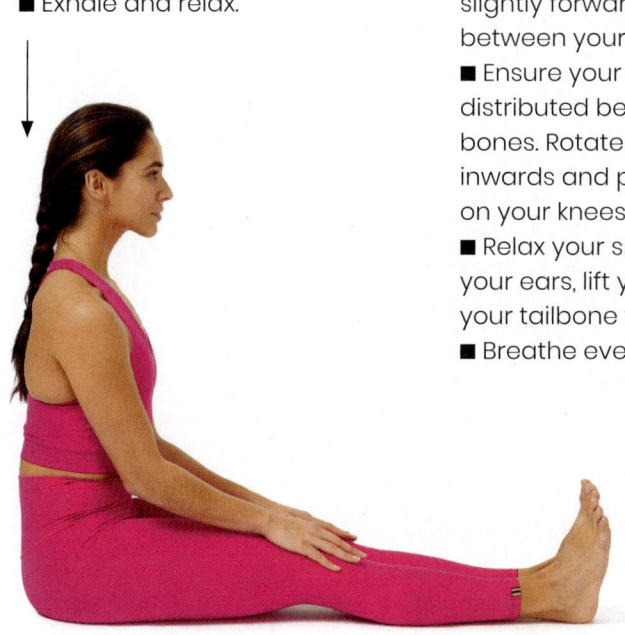

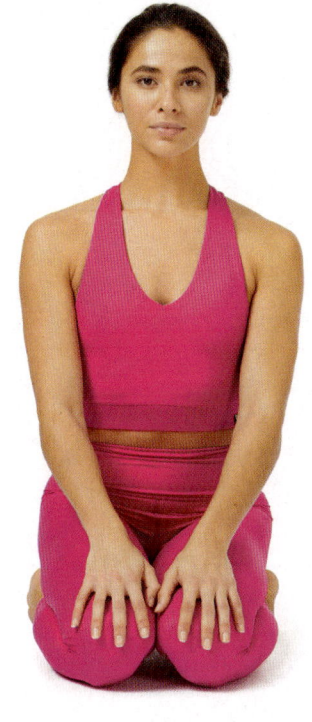

HERO
Virasana

The starting pose for many floor-based yoga postures, Hero opens your hips, relieves back pain and aids digestion.

■ Kneel with your inner knees together, the tops of your feet flat on the floor. Angle your big toes slightly inwards.
■ Exhale and, with your torso slightly forwards, sit back down between your feet.
■ Ensure your weight is evenly distributed between your sitting bones. Rotate your thighs inwards and place your palms on your knees.
■ Relax your shoulders down from your ears, lift your chest and draw your tailbone towards the floor.
■ Breathe evenly.

EASY POSE
Sukhasana

You don't need to sit in Lotus pose to do yoga. Easy pose is grounding, calming and soothes your nervous system.

■ Sit with your legs crossed at your shins (or where comfortable for you).
■ Adjust the fleshy part of your bottom, rooting your sitting bones into the floor.
■ Flex your feet and place your hands either side of your hips, in your lap or on your knees.
■ Draw your navel to your spine and lengthen up out of your pelvis.
■ Relax your shoulders down, open your chest and lengthen your spine and the back of your neck.
■ Breathe evenly into your abdomen.

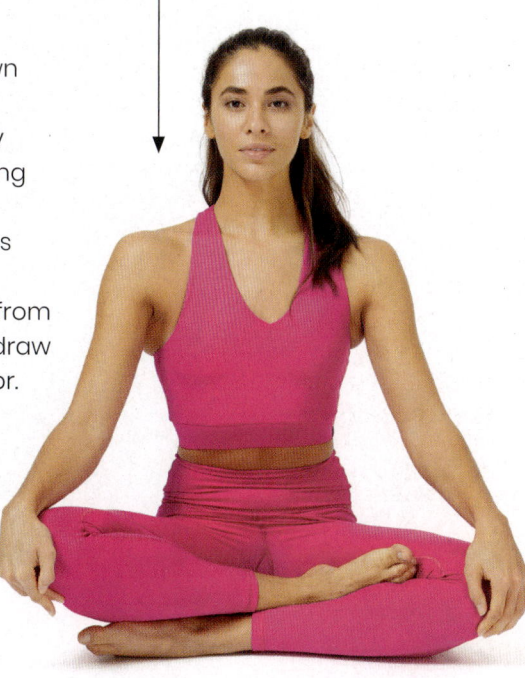

Tips FOR MORNING YOGA

Hitting the mat first thing is easy, if you try these simple ideas

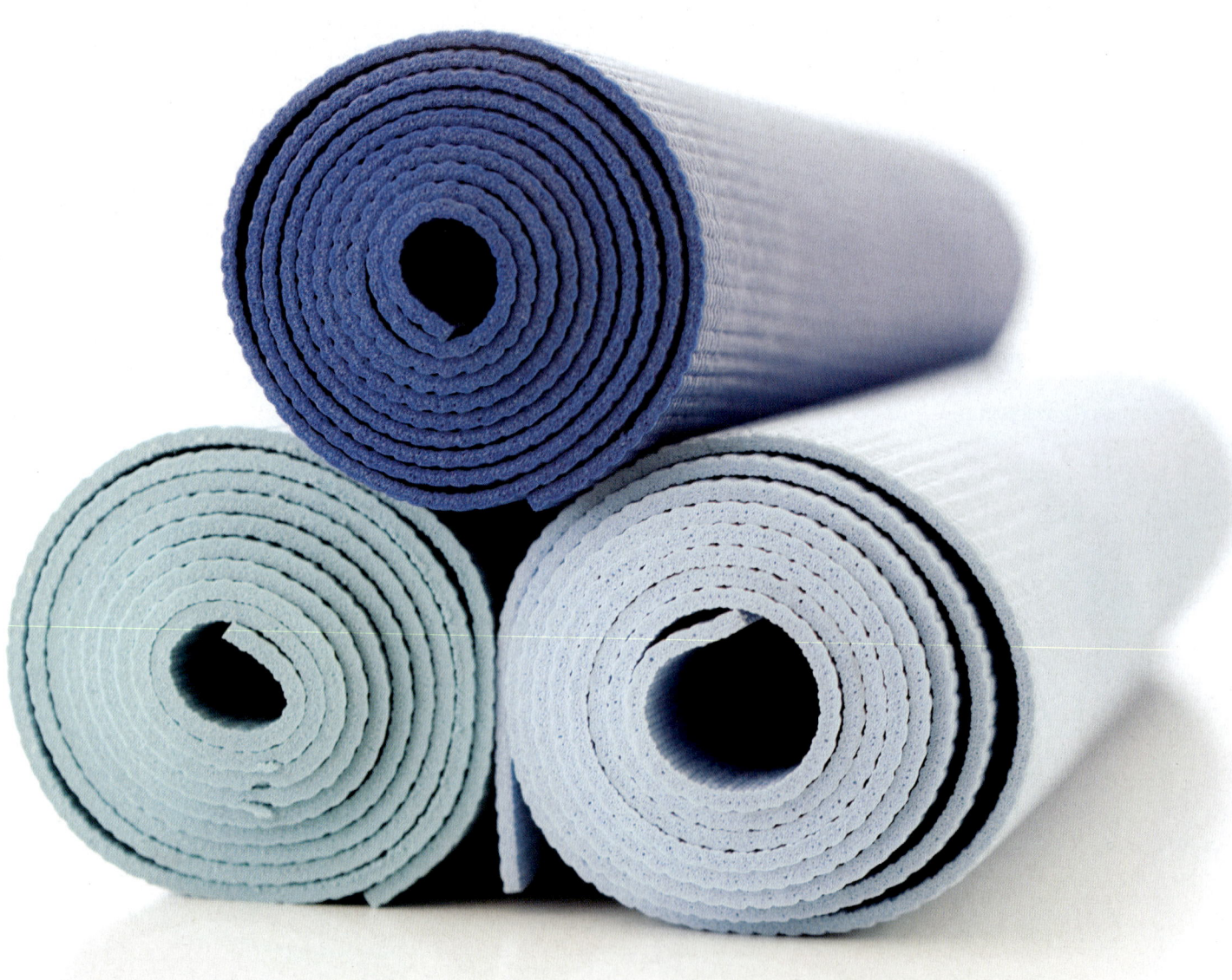

Before you start

If you're new to morning yoga, you may be wondering how on earth you'll fit it into your routine. After all, mornings are often the most hectic time of day as you rush to shower, make breakfast and prepare for work. But, worry not, there are simple strategies you can employ to make your mornings run smoother so you'll have plenty of 'me' time to practise yoga. You'll soon start to feel calmer, less stressed and more organised.

1 Plan ahead
At the start of each week, decide in advance when you're going to practise yoga and schedule the sessions in your diary. This will help you stick to your goals and create a new morning routine. Whether you decide to practise on waking or after you've got the children to school, there's no right or wrong time – just choose whenever suits you best.

2 Set the scene
The great thing about yoga is you can practise it anywhere – all you need is a mat! However, creating a dedicated space can help you experience a deeper, more meditative practice. Find a quiet, uncluttered place in your home with enough space to move and where you won't be disturbed. Ideally, choose a room with a window or other source of natural daylight to help energise your sessions and lift your mood. If that's not possible, use soft lighting or a candle. If the weather is fine, you could even take your practice outside into your garden or a quiet local park.

OPEN A WINDOW DURING YOUR PRACTICE – THE FRESH AIR WILL OXYGENATE YOUR BODY AND BRAIN.

3 Be prepared
Save time searching for your yoga kit every morning by making sure it's always ready for your session. During your practice, keep any props (p35) you'll need to hand – for instance, a block or strap, plus a blanket in case you get cold during relaxation and meditation. You don't need to wear any fancy yoga clothes, just comfortable layers that you can move freely in.

4 Stay hydratated
Start your day with a glass of water or warm water and lemon to rehydrate your body and wake up your metabolism. Avoid drinking too much liquid straight before or during your class as it will sit heavily on your stomach. Yogis believe it also extinguishes your inner fire. If you feel thirsty during your session, take small sips of water and then rehydrate after you finish.

5 Eat later
You should always leave two hours in between eating a meal and doing yoga, to allow your body time to digest. You'll feel lighter and more comfortable practising on an empty stomach – it's no fun doing challenging poses with a tummy full of food! Plan to have breakfast after you finish your yoga session. If you're feeling too hungry to practise, eat a small snack, such as half a banana, 30 minutes beforehand.

6 Warm up
As with any exercise, it's important to warm up your body before your yoga session. Aim to take your body through all the planes of movement you'll be doing in the class (forwards, backwards, sideways and twisting), focusing on all the main muscle groups you'll be using. Turn to page 96 for a collection of yoga warm-up poses.

7 Listen to your body
As you practise, check in with your body and notice how it's feeling today. Is it stiff and achy, bouncy and energised? Listen to the messages it gives you and tailor your practice accordingly. If your body's feeling stiff, you can stretch more slowly and deeply; if it's feeling energetic, you can choose a more dynamic sequence.

Stay safe

- If you're new to yoga or exercise, always have a health check with your GP to ensure it's safe for you to practise.
- If you're pregnant, check with your GP or nurse that it's safe for you to practise the poses in this book.
- If you experience any sharp or sudden pain while doing a pose, stop and rest. A mild ache during a stretch or deep pose is acceptable and a sign your body's joints are opening.
- If you have high blood pressure, avoid inverted poses such as Downward-facing dog (p62) or Forward bend (p42).

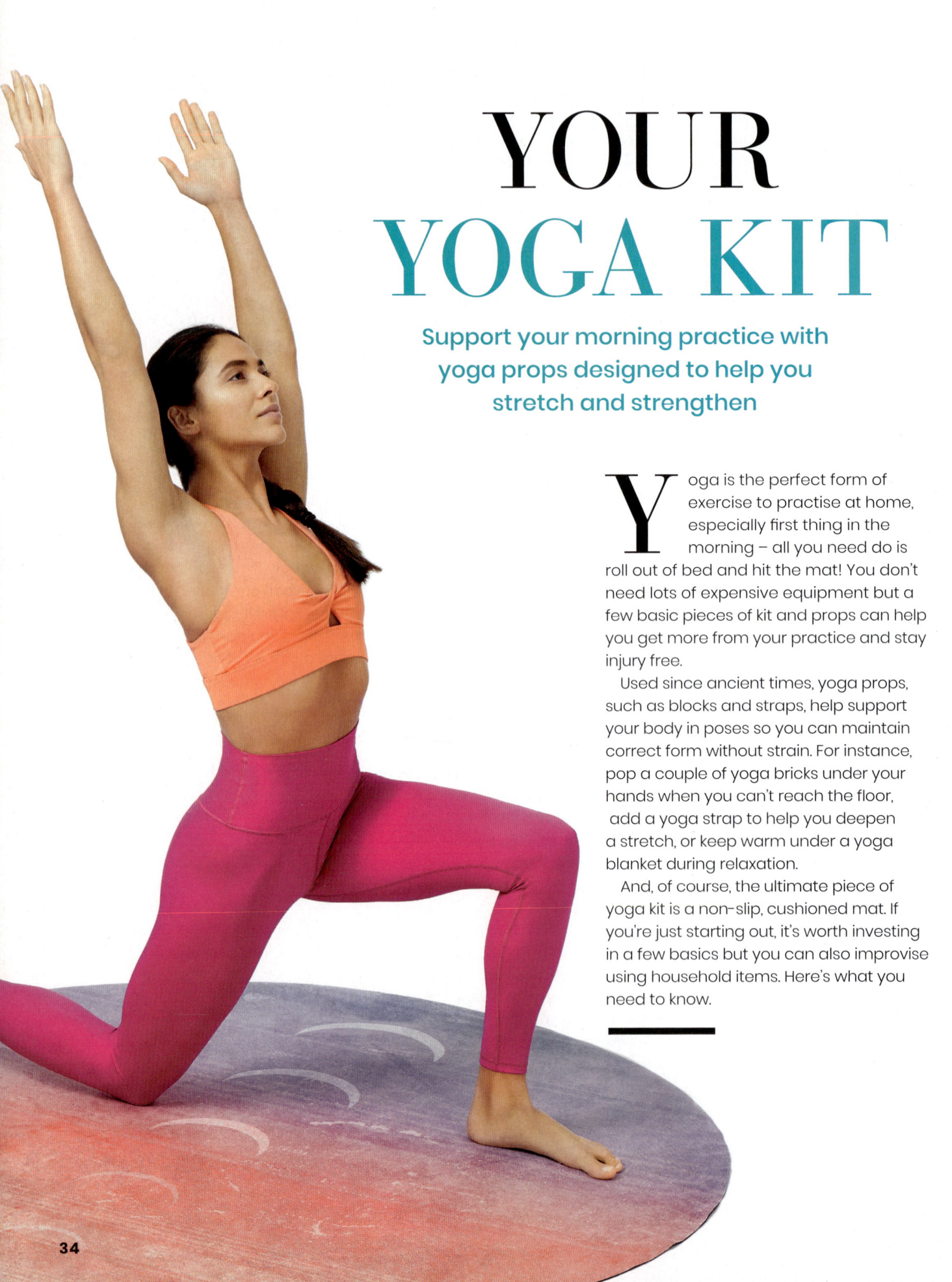

YOUR YOGA KIT

Support your morning practice with yoga props designed to help you stretch and strengthen

Yoga is the perfect form of exercise to practise at home, especially first thing in the morning – all you need do is roll out of bed and hit the mat! You don't need lots of expensive equipment but a few basic pieces of kit and props can help you get more from your practice and stay injury free.

Used since ancient times, yoga props, such as blocks and straps, help support your body in poses so you can maintain correct form without strain. For instance, pop a couple of yoga bricks under your hands when you can't reach the floor, add a yoga strap to help you deepen a stretch, or keep warm under a yoga blanket during relaxation.

And, of course, the ultimate piece of yoga kit is a non-slip, cushioned mat. If you're just starting out, it's worth investing in a few basics but you can also improvise using household items. Here's what you need to know.

Props

Block

Do you find it hard sitting up straight in Staff pose (p30) or Cross-legged pose (p30)? Slip a foam block under your bottom to bring your back into alignment, take the pressure off your hips and sit more comfortably. You can also use a block as a support for your head during Corpse pose (p92) or for your hands if they don't reach the floor during standing poses such as Wide-legged forward bend (p54). A block is slightly flatter and wider than a brick. If you don't have one, you can use a packet of printer paper instead.

Blanket

Keep a blanket or two handy during your yoga sessions. Folded up, they can provide a useful support for your back in inverted poses. Or roll them up and pop under your heels if they won't reach the floor in poses such as Garland (p60) or under your neck or knees during Corpse pose (p92). A blanket is also handy to keep you warm during relaxation when your body temperature starts to fall. Lay a blanket over you during Corpse pose or use it like a shawl when sitting cross-legged for meditation (p122). Any blanket will do but yoga blankets are ideal.

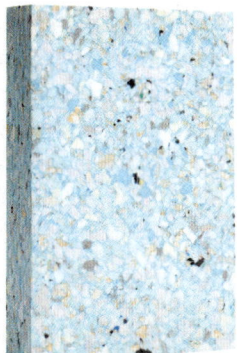

+ Yogamatters Chipped Foam Yoga Block (£5/$6.50; yogamatters.com)

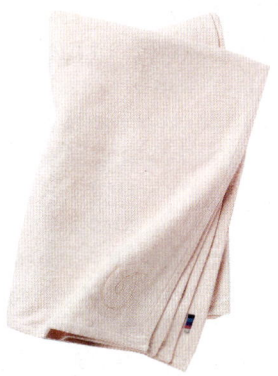

+ Yogamatters Organic Cotton Yoga Blanket (£26/$34; yogamatters.com)

MORNING MATS

Inspire your yoga practice with these uplifting, eco-friendly yoga mats

< Escape to the ocean on this eco-friendly, sweat-proof mat made from natural tree rubber and recycled polyester. **The Swell (£85/$112; palmsinthewild.com)**

> Breathe in calm on this beautiful grippy mat. An ultra-absorbent microfibre towel layer is bonded to natural tree rubber. It comes with carrying strap. **Yoga Design Lab Breathe Combo Mat (£84/$110; yogadesignlab.com)**

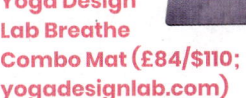

> Stay aligned on this sunny non-slip, cushioned mat, made from eco polyurethane and a natural rubber base. It comes with a mat bag. **Liforme Rainbow Hope Yoga Mat (£135/$178; liforme.com)**

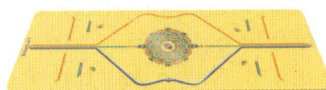

> Enhance your yoga space with this pretty circular yoga mat in Luna Sunrise. It has a sweat-activated, slip-resistant top layer. **eQua eKO Round Yoga Mat 3mm (£79/$104; eu.manduka.com)**

Yoga mat

To practise yoga safely and effectively, you need lots of grip with your hands and feet. A 'sticky' yoga mat is ideal to stop your limbs slipping during poses. It can also provide cushioning for your body during reclining poses and relaxation. Mats come in different levels of thickness and texture so it's worth shopping around to find one that suits you best. You don't have to spend a fortune – there are options for every budget.

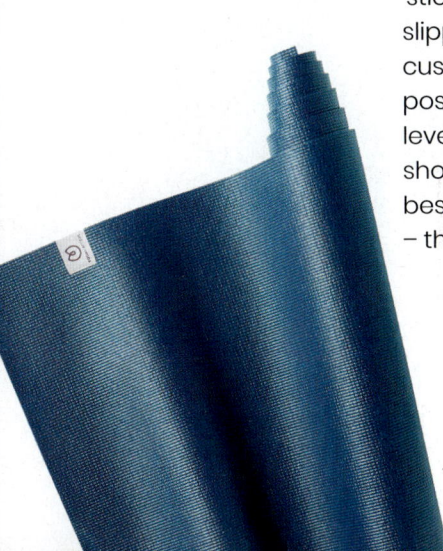

+ Yogamatters Sticky Yoga Mat (£25/$33; yogamatters.co.uk)

Strap

A yoga strap or belt, is handy for lengthening your reach in poses and helping you stretch while keeping the correct alignment. Think of it as an extension to your limbs. If you have tight shoulders, hold a strap with both hands in the final stage of Cow face pose (p84). Or if you find it hard to reach your toes in Reclining head-to-toe pose (p90) or Dancer pose (p58), loop a strap around the arch of your foot and hold it with both hands. If you don't have a strap, try using a belt.

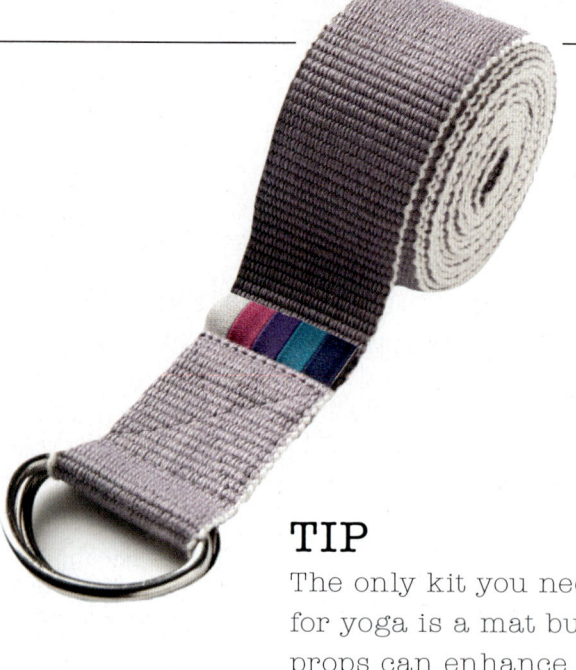

TIP
The only kit you need for yoga is a mat but props can enhance your practice.

+ Yogamatters Organic Cotton D-ring Yoga Belt (£8/$10.50; yogamatters.com)

Brick

Usually made of foam or cork, a yoga brick is a great multi-tasking tool for your yoga sessions. It can support parts of your body, such as your hands, head or back during practice. It's also ideal for modifying more challenging poses if you're a beginner, injured or simply find it hard to reach the floor. For instance, pop one under your forearms during Lizard pose (p70). A brick also adds a challenge to a pose, for instance, place one between your thighs during Chair pose (p44) to work your thigh muscles. If you don't have a yoga brick, try using a small, thick hardcover book.

Meditation cushion

One of the secrets of meditation is to ensure you're comfortable and supported. If you're sitting cross-legged, raising your hips above your knees will ensure your spine stays straight. A cushion filled with natural buckwheat will mould to your body, allowing it to release and relax into meditation. You can adjust the height by removing or adding the filling. Improvise with a firm cushion or rolled up yoga mat or blanket.

Bolster

Soft but supportive, a cylindrical bolster is the ultimate tool for yoga relaxation sessions. Pop one under your knees in Corpse pose (p92) to ease a stiff lower back. Place one on the floor to rest your head in Wide-legged forward bend (p54) or Child's pose (p86). It's also great to support you when you're lounging on the floor. If you don't have a yoga bolster, try using a firm pillow or two, or thick, rolled up blankets.

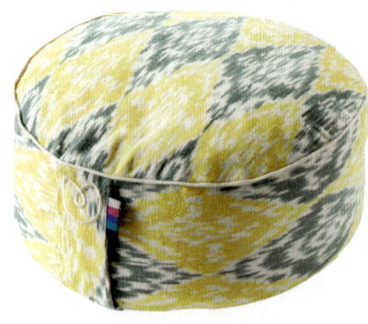

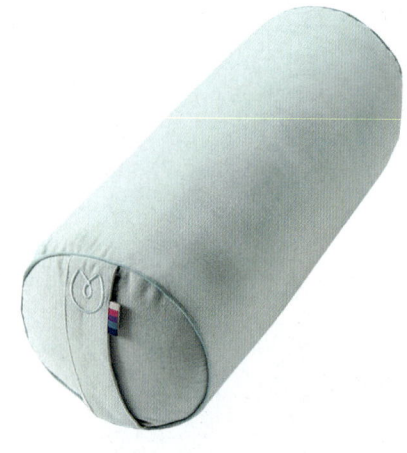

+ Yogamatters Yoga Brick (£7/$9; yogamatters.com)

+ Yogamatters Spring Ikat Round Buckwheat Meditation Cushion (£35/$46; yogamatters.com)

+ Yogamatters Organic Cotton Buckwheat Bolster (£40/$53; yogmatters.com)

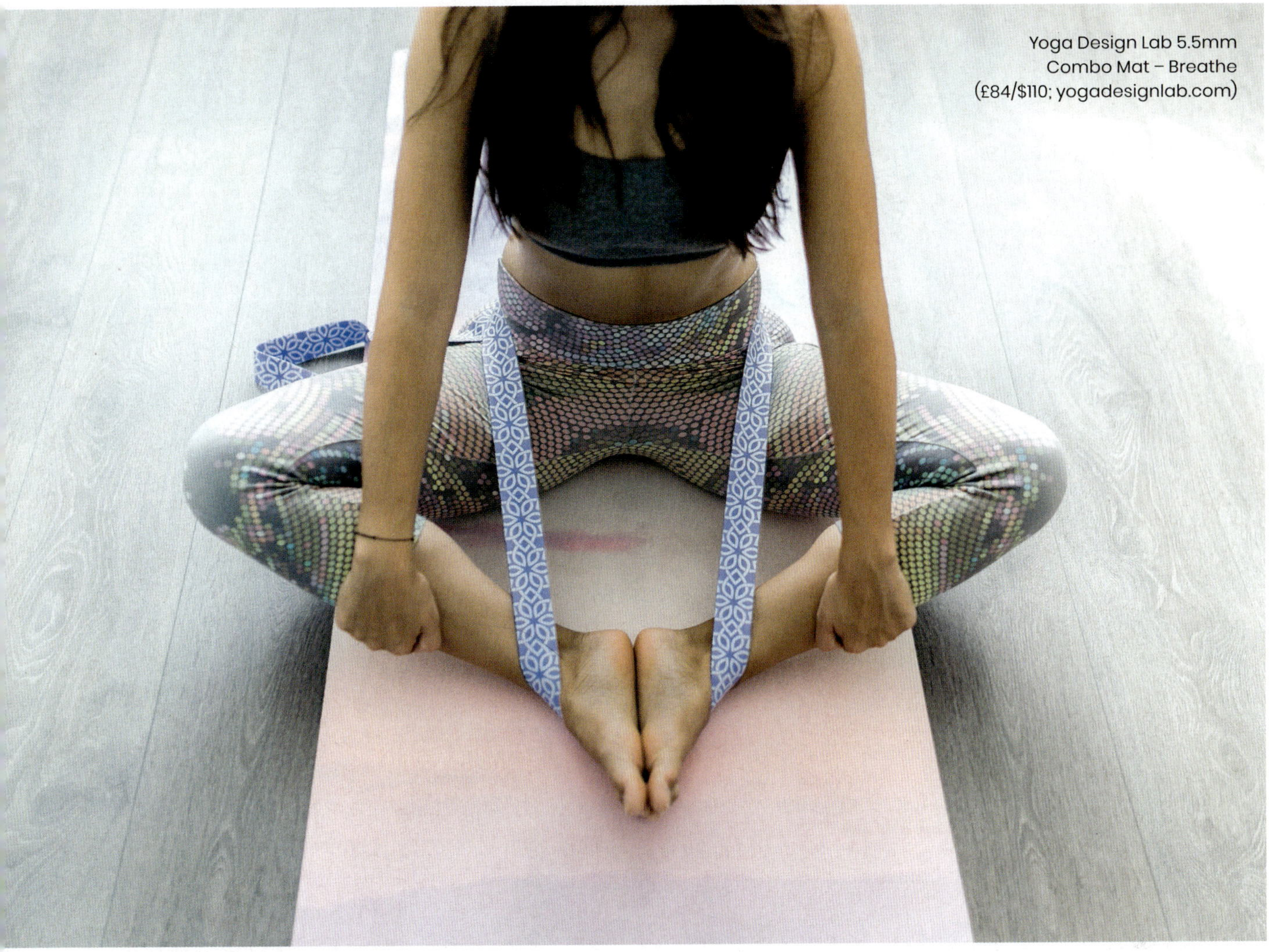

Props

Yoga Design Lab 5.5mm Combo Mat – Breathe (£84/$110; yogadesignlab.com)

Handy helpers

Enhance your morning sessions with a few mindfulness tools

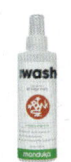

Mat cleaner
Keep your mat clean and fresh with an all-natural, sanitising spray. This Manduka Energising Gingergrass Mat Wash (€15; eu.manduka.com) is full of zingy ginger and lavender essential oils.

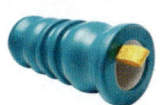

Muscle roller
Boost your relaxation and recovery with a foam roller. This Manta Foam Roller (£37.99/$50; mantahealth.com), designed by an osteopath, has a groove that follows the contours of your spine.

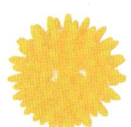

Foot massager
Treat your hard-working hands and feet with a DIY massage ball. This Spikey Massage Ball (£3.95/$5.20; healf.com) eases away aches and boosts circulation.

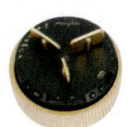

Meditation aid
If you find it hard to relax, Morphée (€79.95; morphee.co) is a clever non-digital device that offers a variety of soothing guided sessions, including body scan, breathing, visualisation and relaxation to help you feel calm.

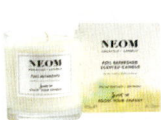

Yoga candle
Light up dark mornings with an uplifting, natural candle. This Neom Feel Refreshed Scented Candle (£35/$46; neomorganics.com) is fragranced with 24 oils, including lemon and basil.

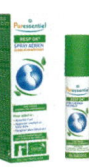

Room spray
Did you know incense can cause indoor air pollution? Swap it for a purifying aromatherapy spray such as this Puressentiel Respiratory Spray (£9.99/$13; uk.puressentiel.com).

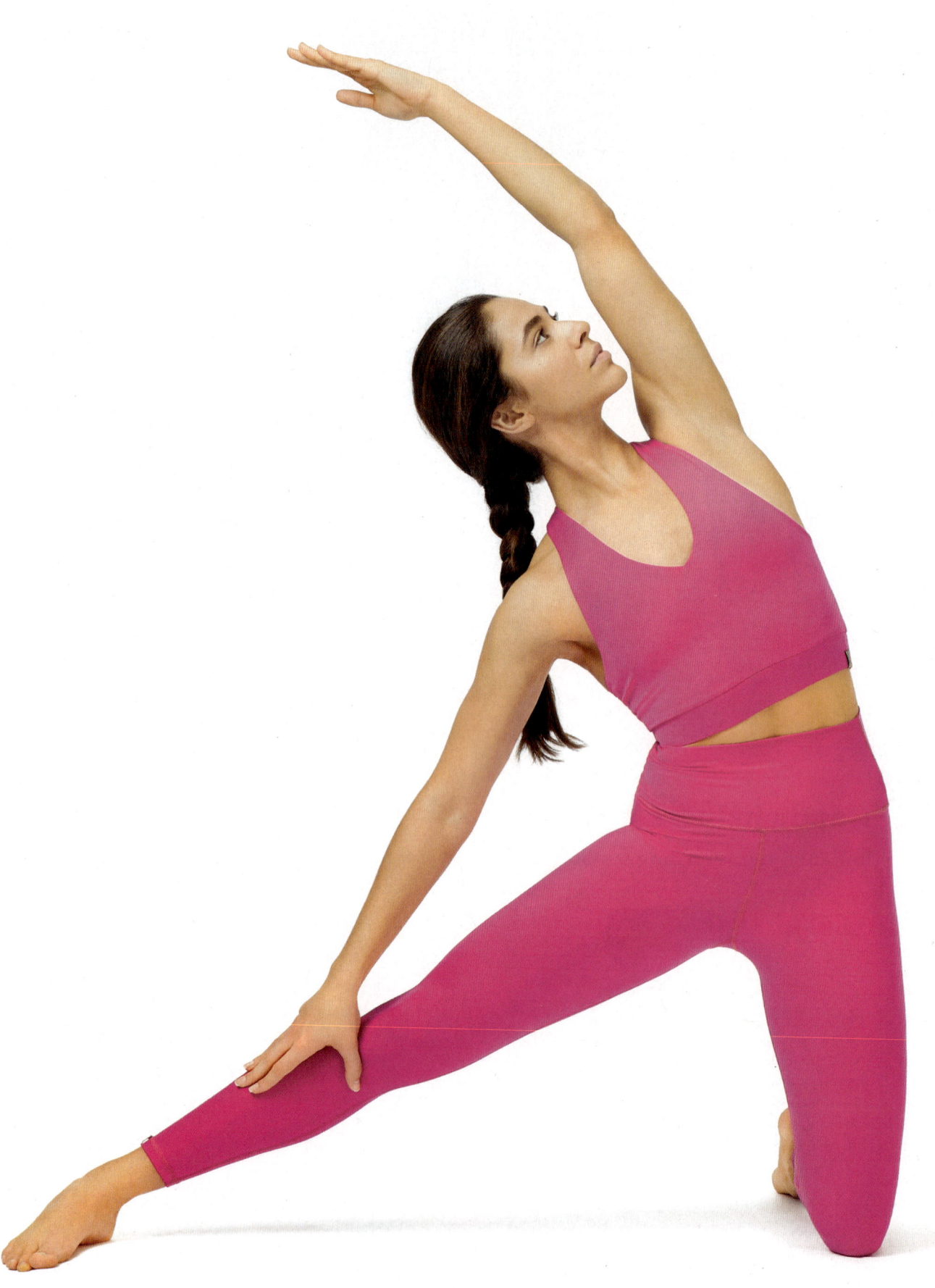

THE POSES

Ready to start practising morning yoga? In this section, you'll find a collection of yoga poses specially designed to wake up your body and mind, boost your energy and get you focused for the day ahead. Each pose comes with step-by-step instructions and modifications; read these carefully before trying the poses. Once you've got the hang of them, you can select a few poses to suit your daily needs – or try the tailored sequences featured in the next chapter.

MOUNTAIN POSE
Tadasana

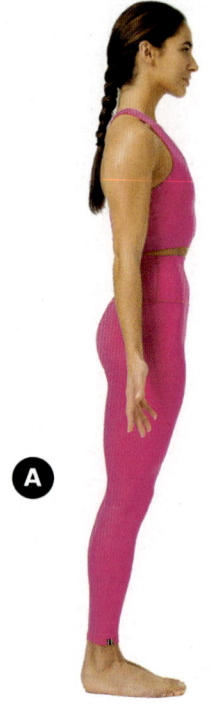

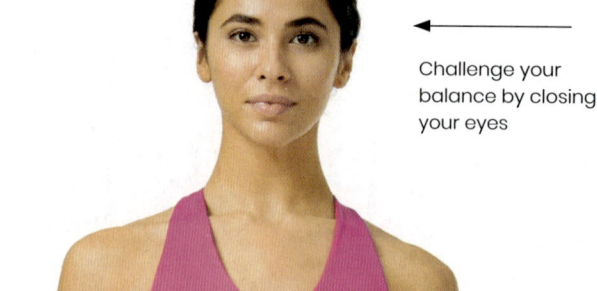

Challenge your balance by closing your eyes

- Stand with your feet together and parallel. Balance your weight evenly over each foot, spread your toes and root into the floor through your big and little toes.
- Lift the inner arches of your feet by drawing your ankles away from each other.
- Keep your knees over your ankles and your pelvis over your knees.
- Relax your bottom and let your tailbone release to the floor. Breathe deeply and evenly.
- Draw your navel towards your spine and relax your shoulders down your back.
- Let your arms hang by your sides and gently extend through to your fingertips. Release and lengthen the back of your neck (A).
- Inhale, ground through your feet and lengthen through to the crown of your head, keeping your shoulders down and maintaining the length in your torso when you exhale. Continue to breathe gently, feeling a sense of grounding on each out breath.
- Rest in the pose for up to 20 to 30 seconds.

TIP
Mountain pose is the starting position for most standing poses. But it's a beneficial pose to practise by itself, too.

Benefits
+ Calms your mind
+ Improves your posture
+ Strengthens your spine, legs and feet

/Standing poses

EXTENDED MOUNTAIN POSE
Urdhva hastasana

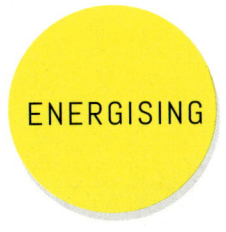
ENERGISING

VARIATION

- Begin in Mountain pose (p40).
- Inhale and root though your feet as you lift your waist out of your hips to lengthen your spine. At the same time, turn your palms outwards and stretch your arms to the sides and overhead.
- Exhale and draw your shoulders down your spine. Engage your leg muscles and draw your navel to your spine (A).
- On each inhale, root down through your feet and lift through your crown and fingertips. On each exhale, visualise your breath travelling down your body and through your feet.
- Keep your gaze soft and stay in the pose for five to 10 deep breaths.

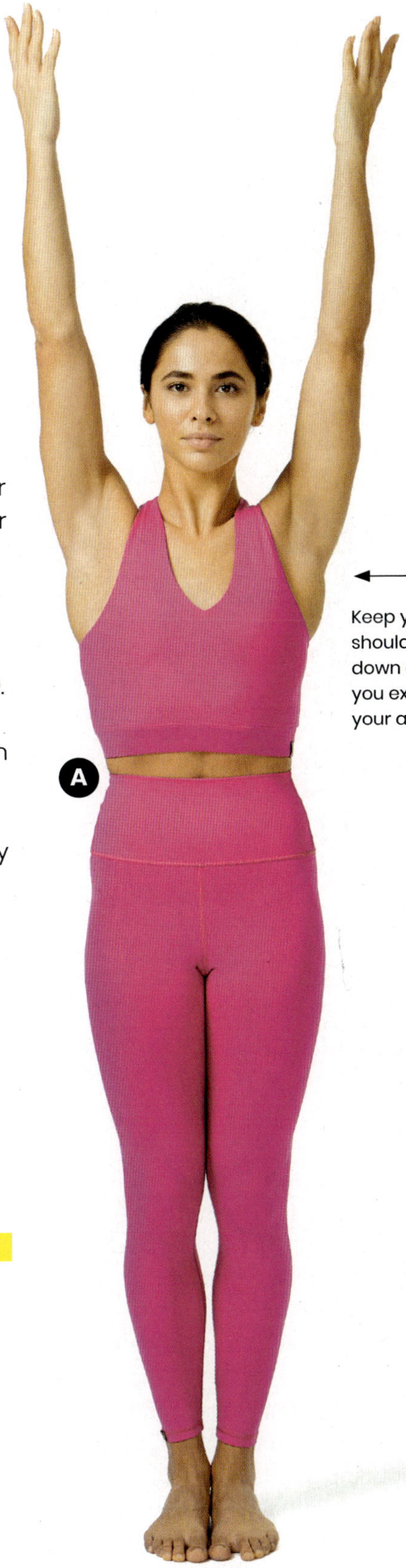

Keep your shoulders down as you extend your arms

Benefits

+ Energises your body and mind
+ Stretches your arms and shoulders
+ Deepens your breath
+ Improves your balance

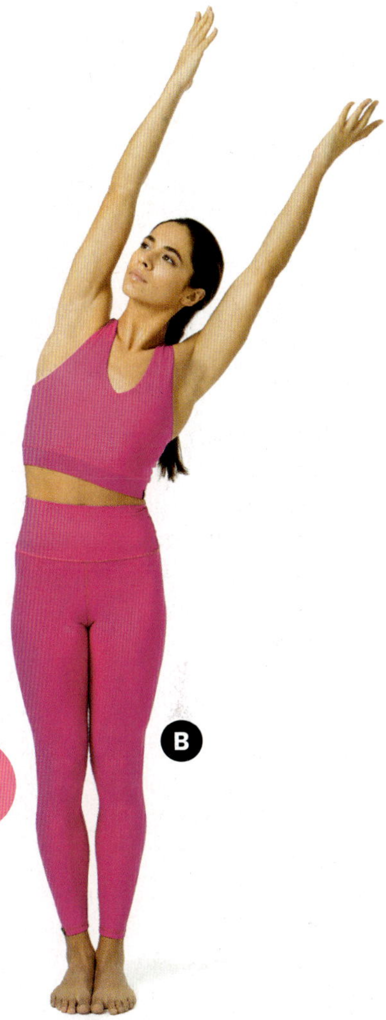

Stretch it out
- For a deep side stretch, from Extended Mountain pose (A), exhale and reach both arms over to your left, feeling the stretch in your right side. Keep your body in one plane, don't bend your torso forwards or backwards (B). Take two to three breaths, then inhale back to upright.
- Repeat on the other side.

STANDING FORWARD BEND
Uttanasana

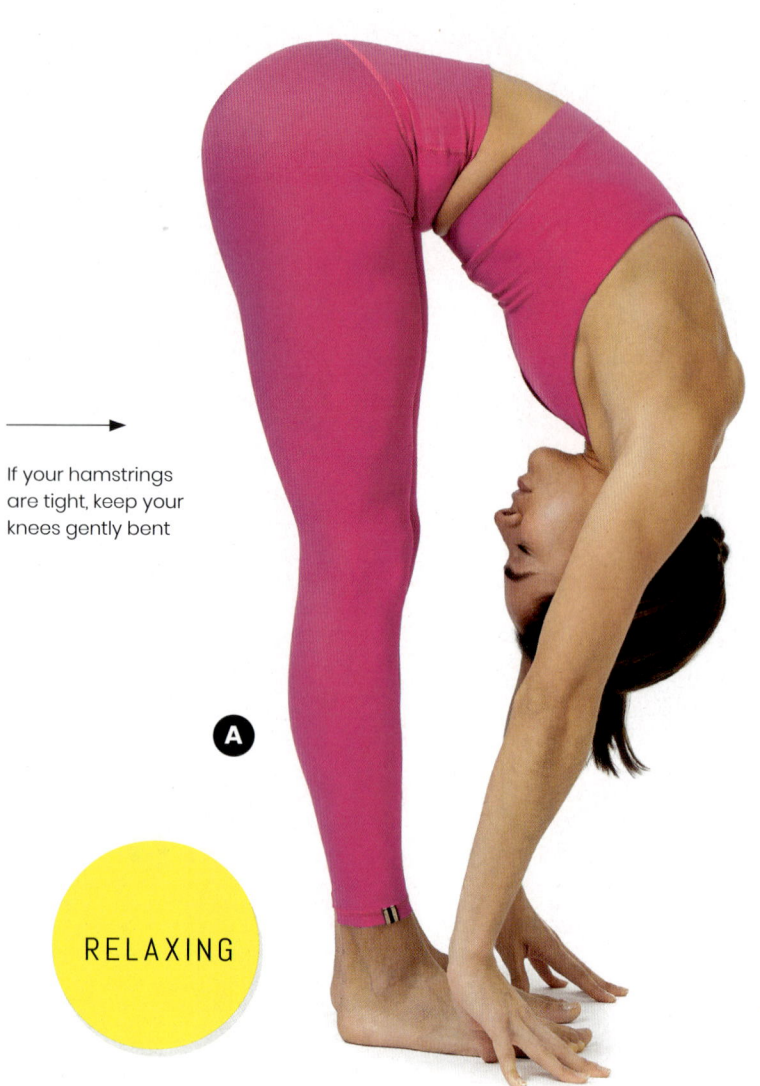

If your hamstrings are tight, keep your knees gently bent

A

RELAXING

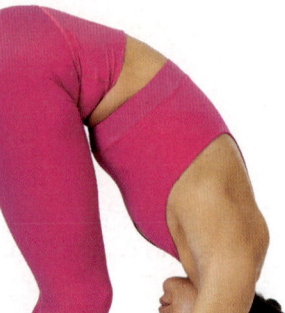

VARIATION

B

Boost your energy
To revitalise your body try Ragdoll pose. Begin in Standing forward bend (A). Take your feet hip-width apart and hold each elbow with the opposite hand. Bend your knees to allow your chest to meet your thighs, then gently straighten them again. Shift your weight forwards and lift your tailbone up (B). Sway from side to side and relax your neck and face, releasing any tension.

- From Mountain pose (p40), inhale and lift your arms up over your head.
- Exhale and fold forwards from your hips. Slowly release your body down towards the floor, lengthening through your torso.
- Bring your fingertips or palms down to the floor, next to your feet (A). If your hands don't touch the floor, cross your forearms, holding your elbows.
- Breathe evenly. On each exhale, relax down further, letting go of your upper body and letting your head and arms hang.
- Spend up to one minute in the pose.
- To come out of the pose, inhale and slowly roll upwards, uncurling your spine, one vertebra at a time, until you're in an upright position.

Benefits
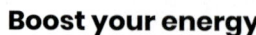

+ Deeply soothing
+ Stretches and strengthens your legs
+ Stretches your spine
+ Relieves fatigue

Standing poses

HALF-STANDING FORWARD BEND
Ardha uttanasana

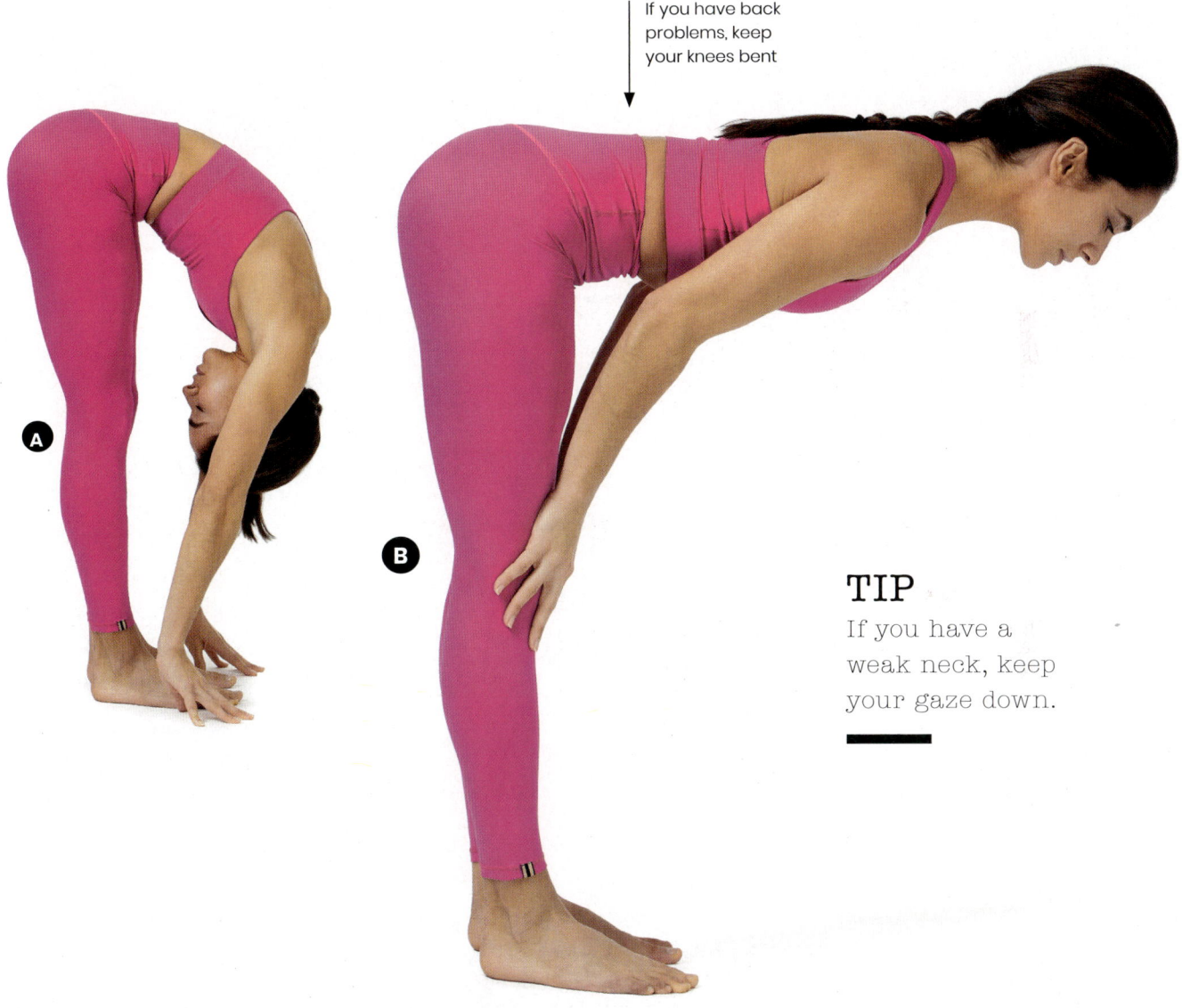

If you have back problems, keep your knees bent

TIP
If you have a weak neck, keep your gaze down.

- Begin in Standing forward bend (p42) (A).
- Press your fingertips into the floor next to your feet.
- Inhale, straighten your elbows and lengthen your crown away from your tailbone. Lift your chest up away from your body to come to a flat back.
- If it's comfortable for your neck, look forwards, keeping your neck long. Root through your hands and feet and draw your shoulder blades down your spine (B).
- Take five deep breaths and release back down to Standing forward bend.

Benefits
+ Strengthens your back
+ Improves your posture
+ Stretches your legs
+ Deeply relaxing

CHAIR POSE
Utkatasana

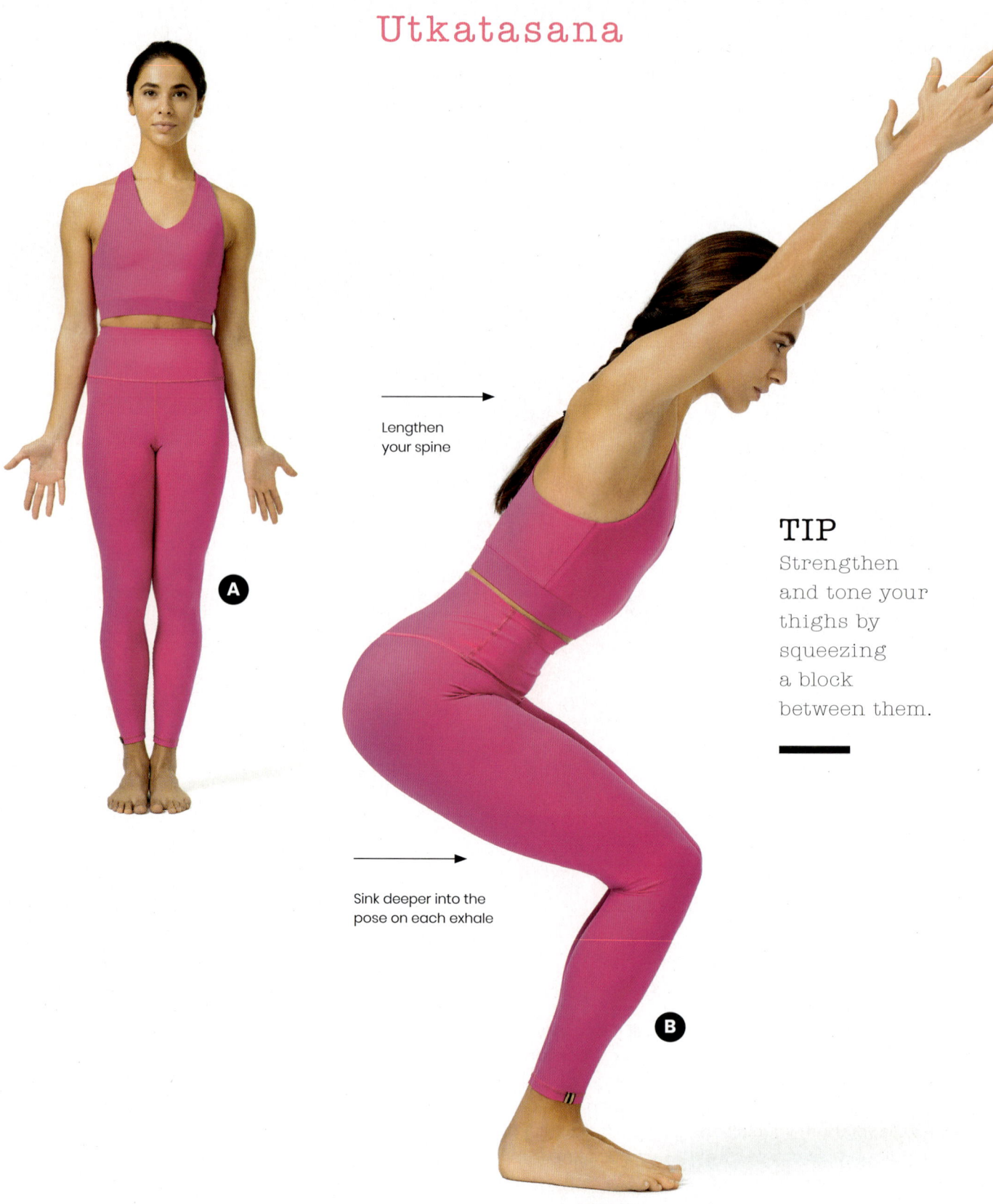

Lengthen your spine

Sink deeper into the pose on each exhale

TIP
Strengthen and tone your thighs by squeezing a block between them.

Standing poses

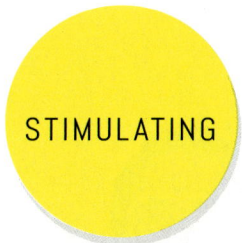
STIMULATING

- Begin in Mountain pose (p40) with your feet together and parallel (A).
- Inhale and stretch your arms over your head with your palms facing inwards and fingers spread.
- As you exhale, bend your knees as if you're sitting down into a chair. Don't let your knees project over your toes.
- Gaze ahead, draw your navel into your spine and relax your shoulders. Lengthen your spine and reach through your hands to your fingertips. Keep your neck in line with your spine (B).
- Take five breaths, lengthening through to your fingertips on an inhale. Sink a little deeper on each exhale.
- To come out of the pose straighten your legs. Repeat the pose three times.

Benefits

+ Tones your arms and legs
+ Strengthens your spine
+ Improves your core strength
+ Stimulates your heart

VARIATION

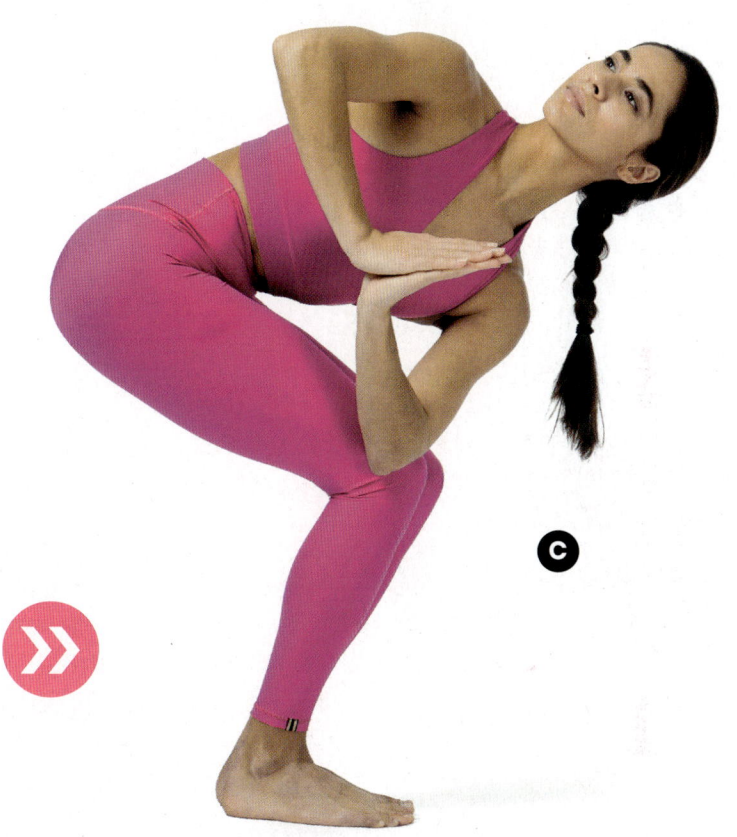

Detox your body
To stretch your spine and aid detoxification, try Revolved chair pose. From Chair pose (B), bring your hands into prayer position at your chest, then inhale and lengthen your spine. Exhale and twist to the right, bringing your left elbow to rest against your outer right thigh. Press your palms together and lever your left arm against your right thigh to deepen the twist, keeping your knees aligned. If comfortable for your neck, turn your gaze upwards (C). Take a few breaths, then return to Chair pose. Repeat on the other side.

TREE
Vrksasana

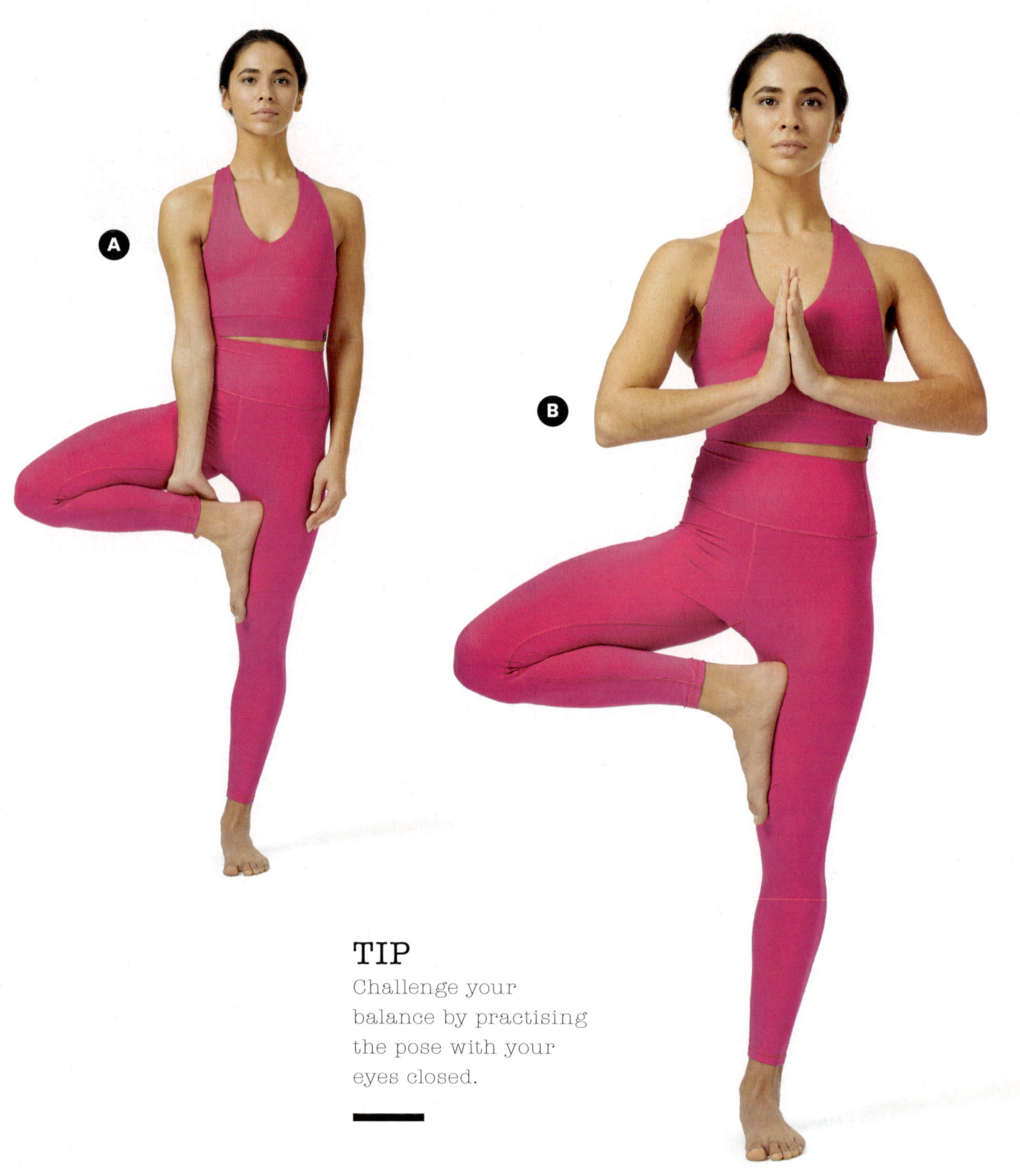

TIP
Challenge your balance by practising the pose with your eyes closed.

Standing poses

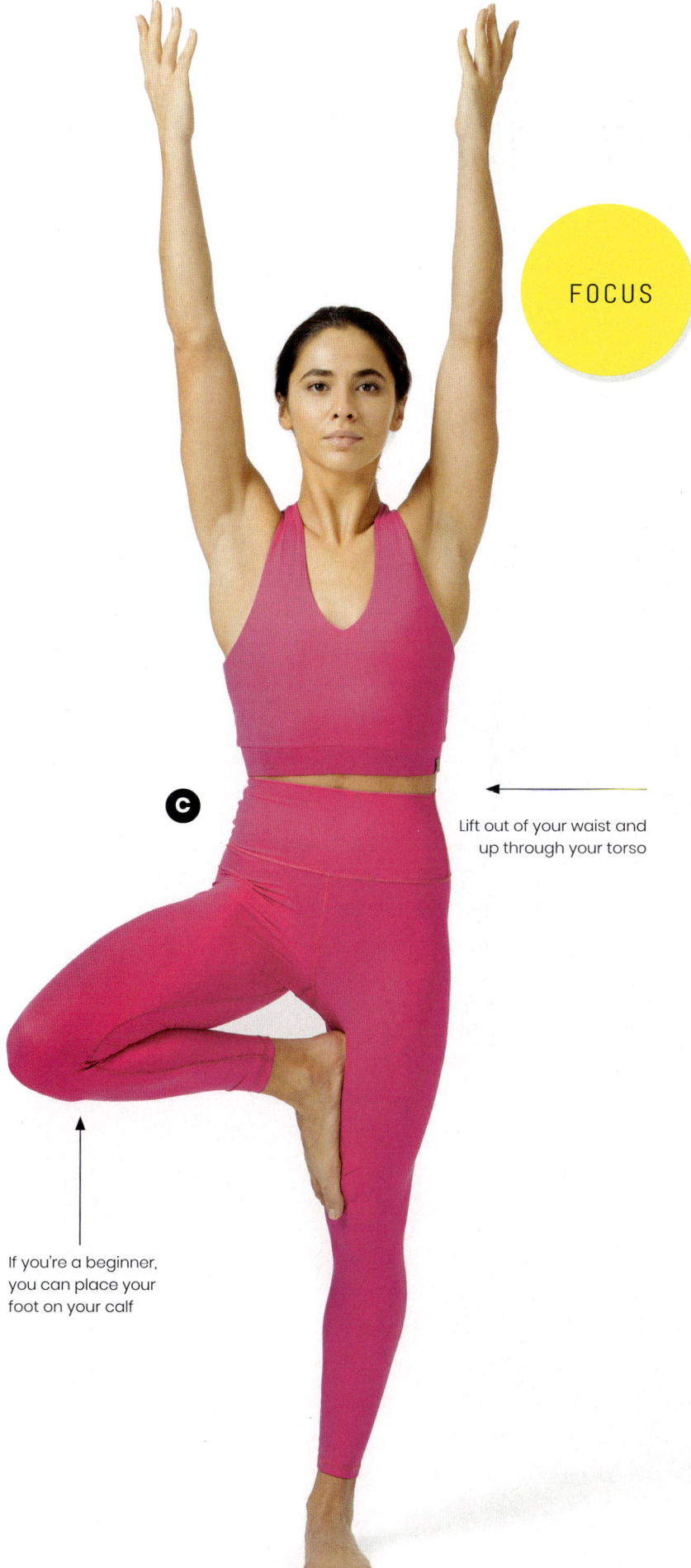

FOCUS

Lift out of your waist and up through your torso

If you're a beginner, you can place your foot on your calf

- From Mountain pose (p40), root your left foot into the ground and carefully transfer your weight onto your left leg.
- Once you feel balanced, keeping a slight bend in your left knee, take your right foot with your right hand and place the inner side of your foot against the inside of your left thigh. To help you balance, set your gaze on a point straight ahead of you.
- Press your foot into your thigh and turn your knee out to the side. Engage your core and release your tailbone towards the floor (A).
- Keeping your shoulders relaxed and your chest lifted, extend your torso out of your waist and up through your crown.
- Slowly bring your hands to Prayer position (B). Stay here for a few breaths.
- If you feel balanced, take your arms overhead with your palms facing each other and parallel. Keep your shoulders relaxed as you extend through your arms to your fingertips (C). Hold for five breaths.
- To come out of the pose, exhale and slowly lower your hands and foot to the start position.
- Repeat on the other side.

Benefits

+ Aids concentration
+ Improves balance
+ Opens your hips and shoulder joints
+ Strengthens your legs

LOW LUNGE
Anjaneyasana

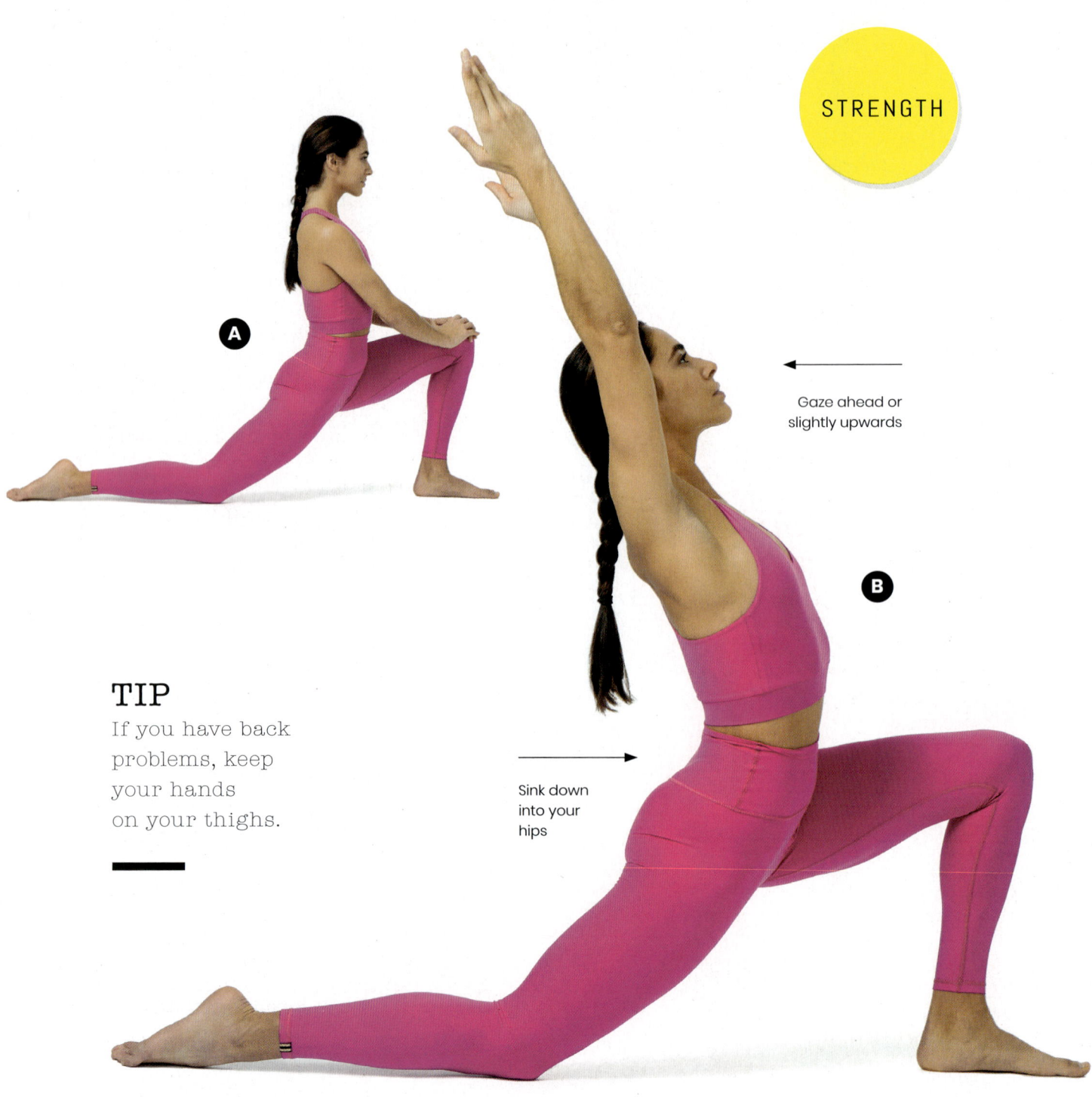

STRENGTH

Gaze ahead or slightly upwards

Sink down into your hips

TIP
If you have back problems, keep your hands on your thighs.

Standing poses

- Start in Mountain pose (p40). Fold forwards from your hips and place your hands either side of your feet, resting on your fingertips.
- Take a large step back with your right leg, resting on the ball of your foot. Lower your right knee to the floor, sliding your foot back until you feel a stretch in your left hip and thigh. Keep your left knee bent over your ankle.
- Keep your hips low and square. Ground through your feet and raise the inner arch of your left foot. Place your hands on your left thigh, take your left hip back and right hip forwards to square them (A).
- Inhale, engage your core and lift your chest up, sweeping your arms up overhead with your palms parallel. Extend your spine out of your pelvis and draw your shoulder blades down your spine. Keep your gaze straight ahead.
- Exhale and, if you feel comfortable, come back into a gentle backbend lifting your gaze up to your hands (B).
- Breathe evenly for five breaths, then exhale, lower your hands and step back into Downward facing dog (p62).
- Repeat on the other side.

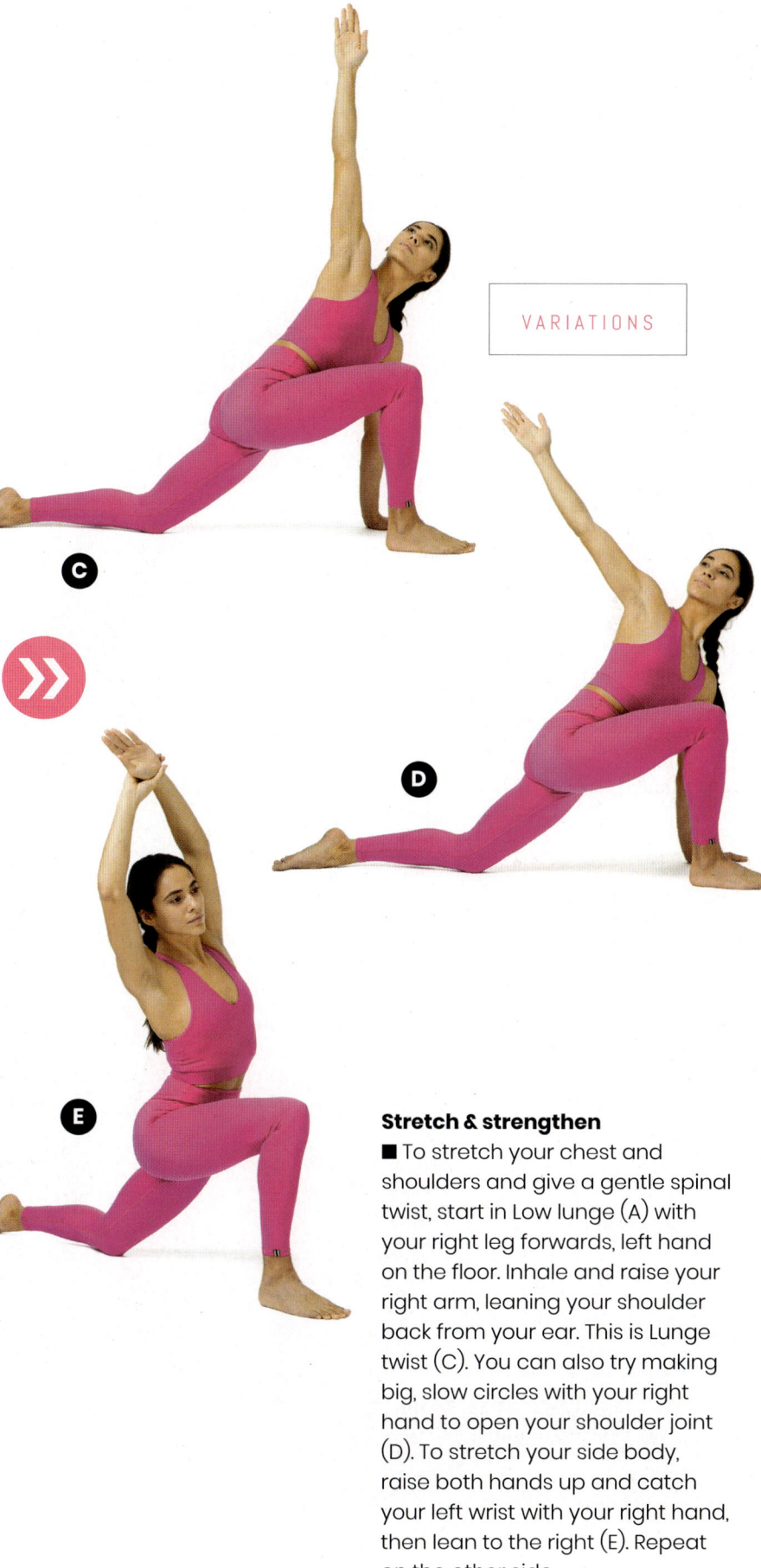

VARIATIONS

Stretch & strengthen
- To stretch your chest and shoulders and give a gentle spinal twist, start in Low lunge (A) with your right leg forwards, left hand on the floor. Inhale and raise your right arm, leaning your shoulder back from your ear. This is Lunge twist (C). You can also try making big, slow circles with your right hand to open your shoulder joint (D). To stretch your side body, raise both hands up and catch your left wrist with your right hand, then lean to the right (E). Repeat on the other side.

Benefits

+ Improves your balance
+ Strengthens your legs and back
+ Stretches your hips and thighs
+ Tones your core

HALF-SPLITS POSE
Ardha hanumanasana

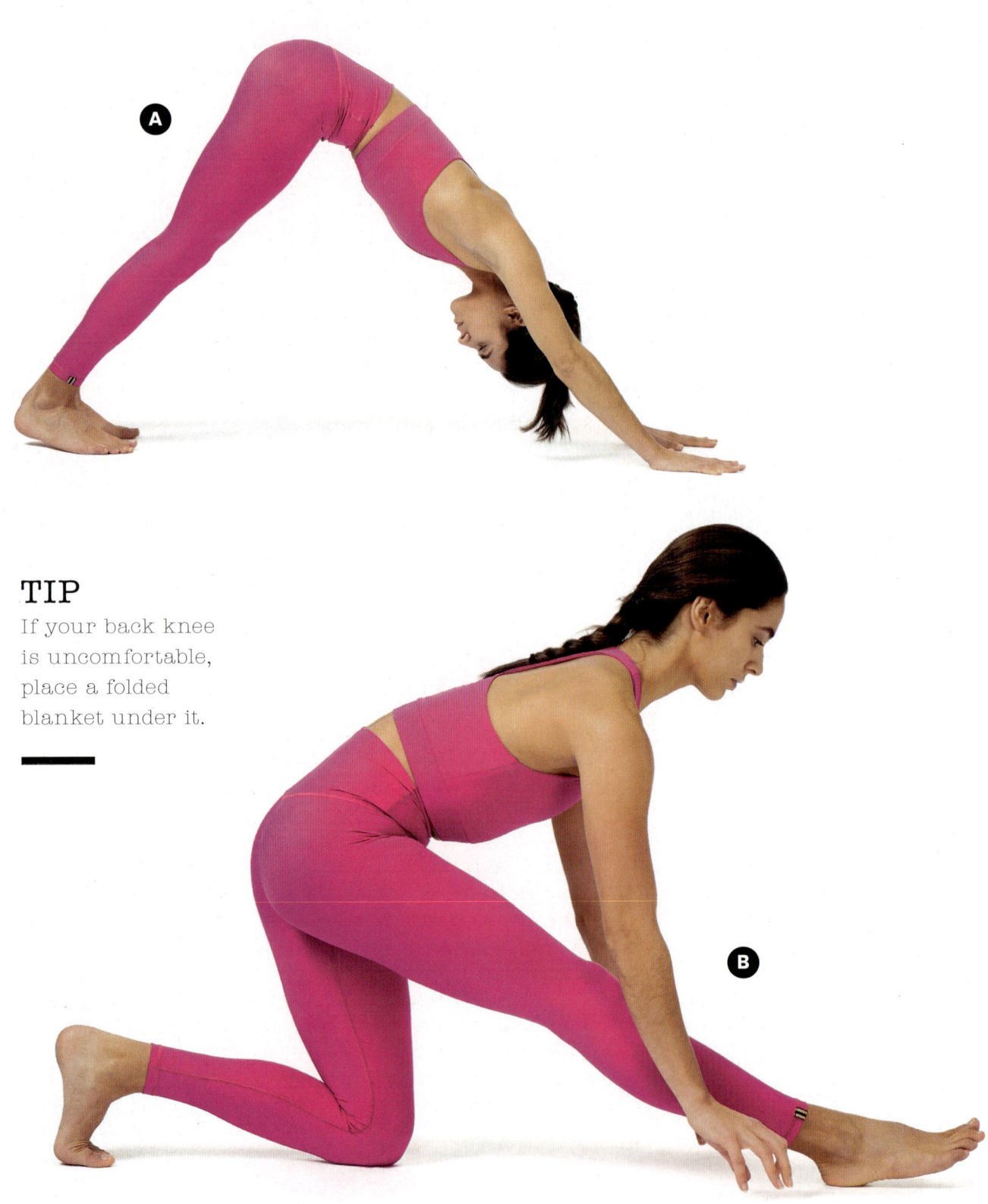

TIP
If your back knee is uncomfortable, place a folded blanket under it.

/ Standing poses

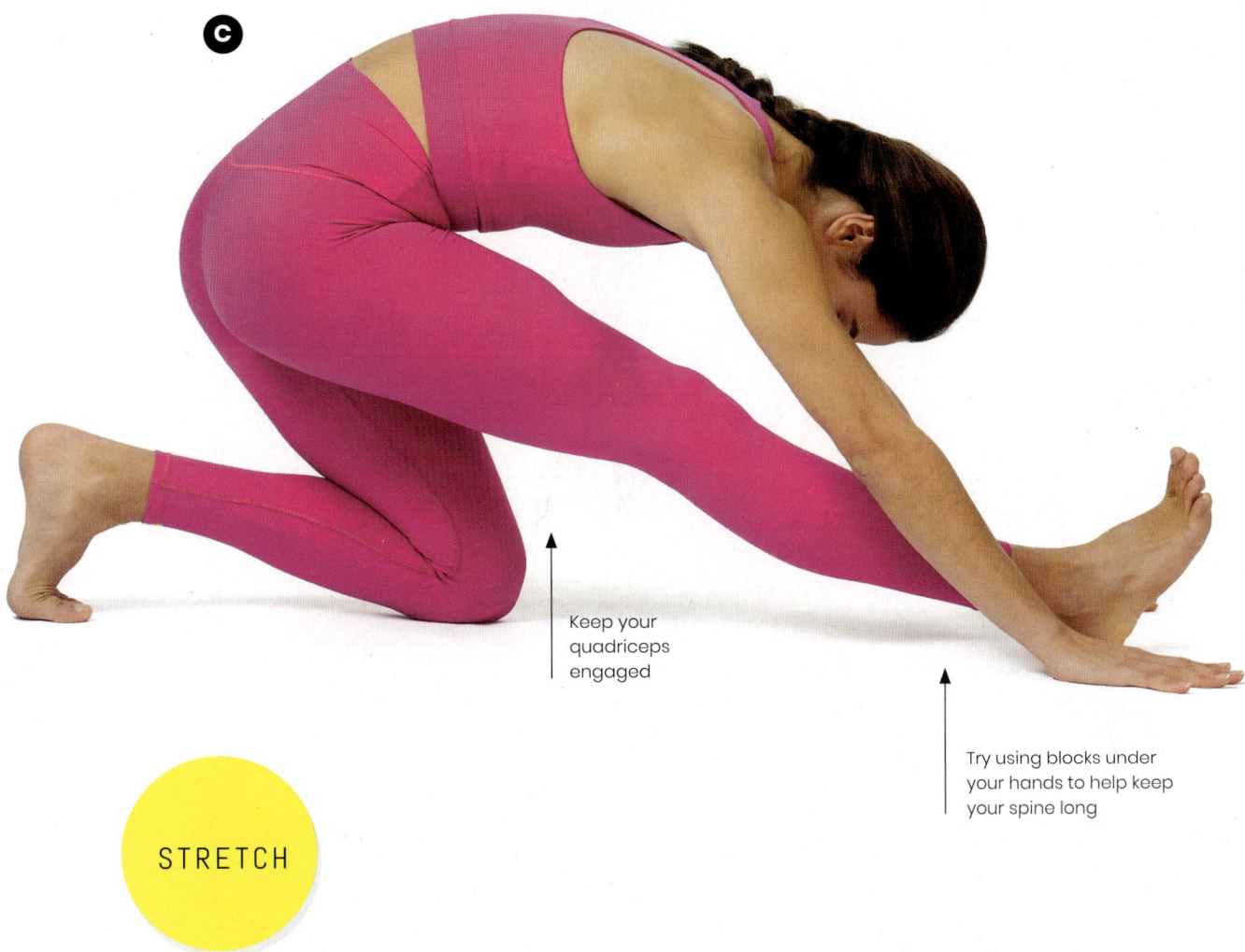

Keep your quadriceps engaged

Try using blocks under your hands to help keep your spine long

STRETCH

- Begin in Downward-facing dog pose (p62) (A).
- Exhale and step your right foot forwards between your hands. Lower down onto your left knee and tuck your left toes under.
- Flex your right foot, coming up onto the heel and extending your toes back towards you while straightening your right leg (B).
- Inhale and lengthen your spine, then exhale and fold your torso over your right leg.
- Keep your hips square and reach your chest forwards. Draw your shoulder blades down your back and away from your ears (C).
- Stay in the pose for five to 10 breaths.
- To come out of the pose, press your palms into the floor and return to Downward-facing dog pose (A).
- Repeat on the other side.

Benefits

+ Stretches your hamstrings and thighs
+ Strengthens your legs
+ Stretches your back
+ Stimulates your digestion

HIGH LUNGE
Alanasana

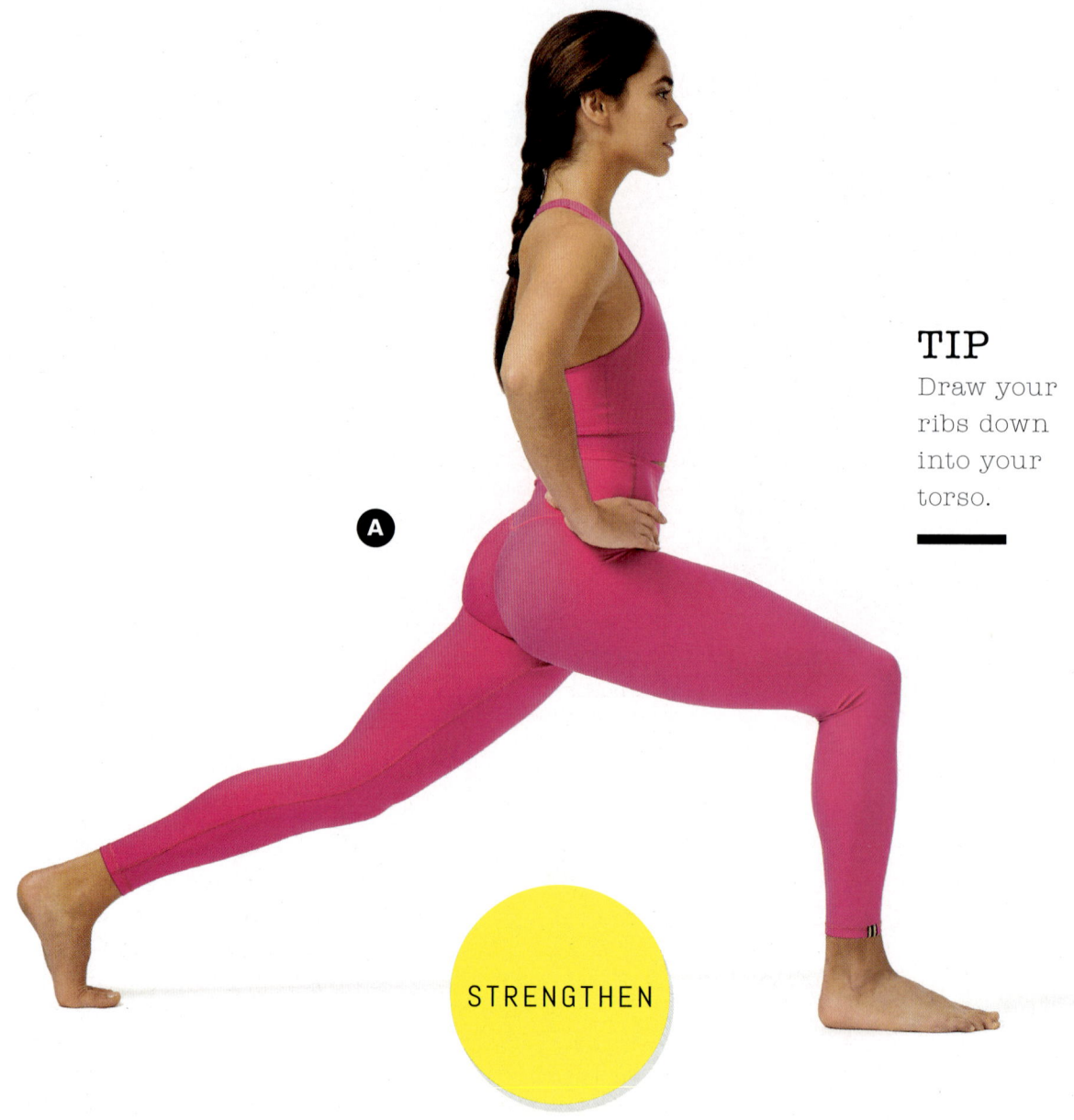

TIP
Draw your ribs down into your torso.

STRENGTHEN

- Start in Mountain pose (p40) with your feet hip-width apart.
- Fold forwards from your hips and place your hands either side of your feet, resting on your fingertips.
- Take a large step straight back with your left leg, to rest on the ball of your foot. Straighten your leg and extend through your left heel. Keep your bent right knee over your right ankle.
- Place your hands on your hips, take your right hip back and your left hip forwards to square your pelvis. Draw your navel to your spine to engage your core (A).
- Inhale and sweep your arms out to the sides and overhead, until your hands are parallel with your palms facing (B).
- Breathe evenly for five deep breaths.
- To come out of the pose, exhale and release your arms, stepping your left foot forwards back into Mountain pose.
- Repeat on the other side.

/ Standing poses

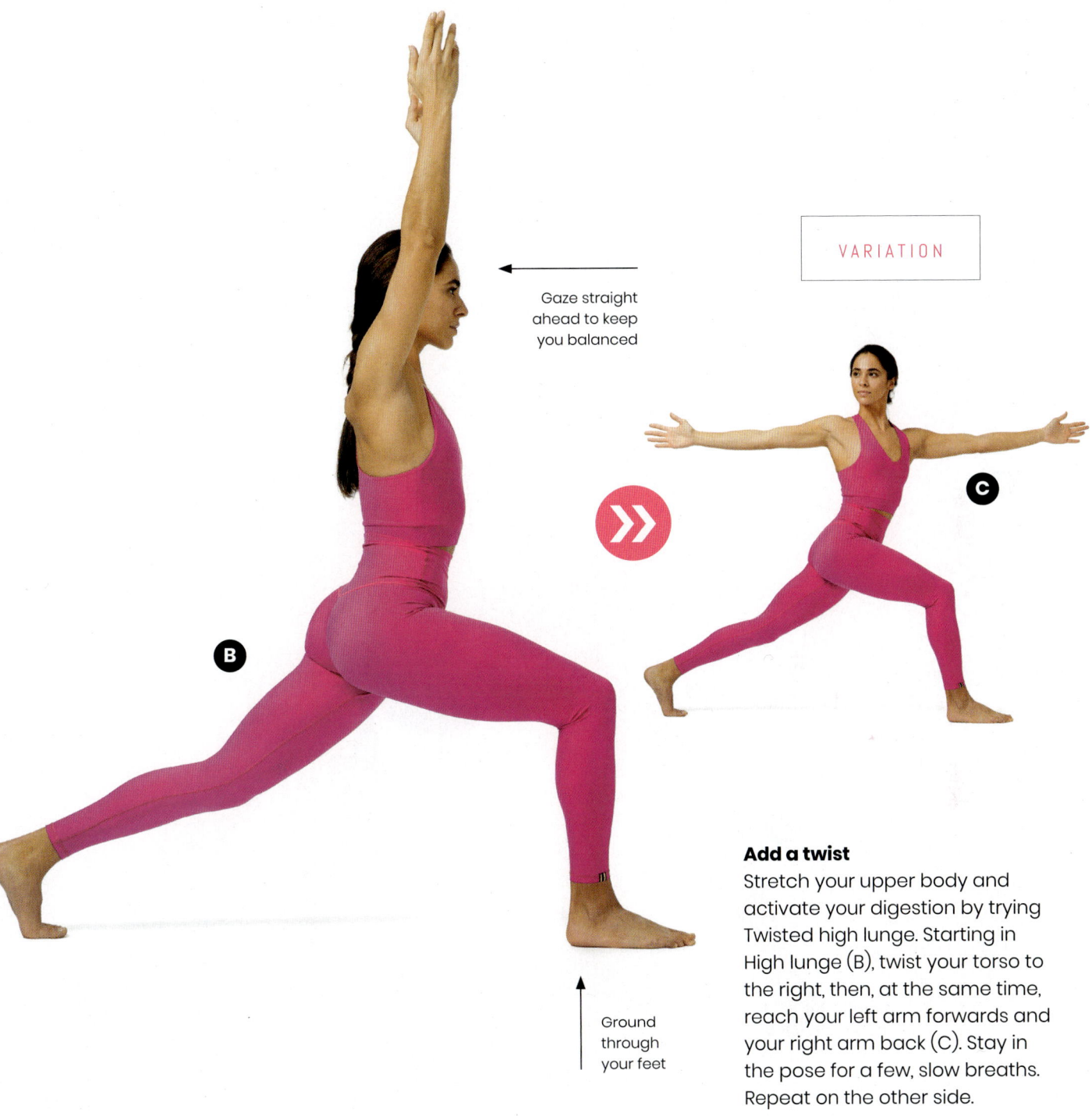

Gaze straight ahead to keep you balanced

VARIATION

Ground through your feet

Add a twist
Stretch your upper body and activate your digestion by trying Twisted high lunge. Starting in High lunge (B), twist your torso to the right, then, at the same time, reach your left arm forwards and your right arm back (C). Stay in the pose for a few, slow breaths. Repeat on the other side.

Benefits

+ Builds stamina
+ Strengthens your legs
+ Energises your mind
+ Releases tight hips

WIDE-LEGGED STANDING FORWARD BEND
Prasarita padottanasana

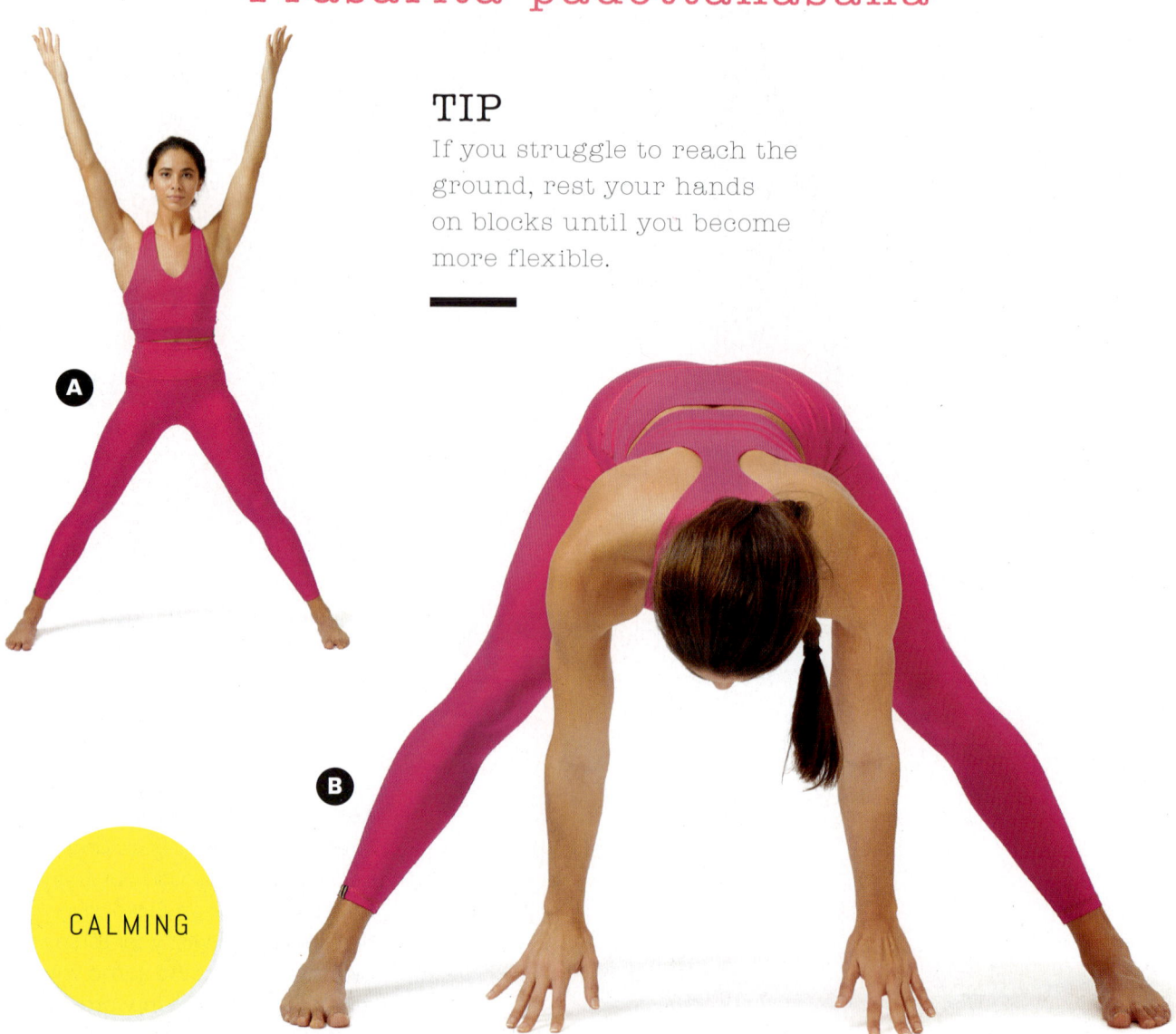

TIP
If you struggle to reach the ground, rest your hands on blocks until you become more flexible.

CALMING

- From Mountain pose (p40), step your feet wide, keeping their inner edges parallel. Lift the inner arches and ground through the outer edges of your feet.
- Inhale and take your arms overhead, extending through your hands and lengthening your spine out of your waist, keeping your shoulders down (A).
- Exhale and fold forwards from your hips keeping your back flat. When your spine is parallel to the floor, bring your hands down to the mat, shoulder-width apart, with your fingers facing forwards (B).
- On each inhale lengthen your spine, on each exhale fold deeper, lowering your head to the floor and letting your neck relax.
- Engage your thighs and, keeping your spine long, let your head and hands relax down as far as is comfortable (C).
- Stay in the pose for up to one minute.
- To come out of the pose, place your hands on your hips and inhale, slowly returning to standing.

/ Standing poses

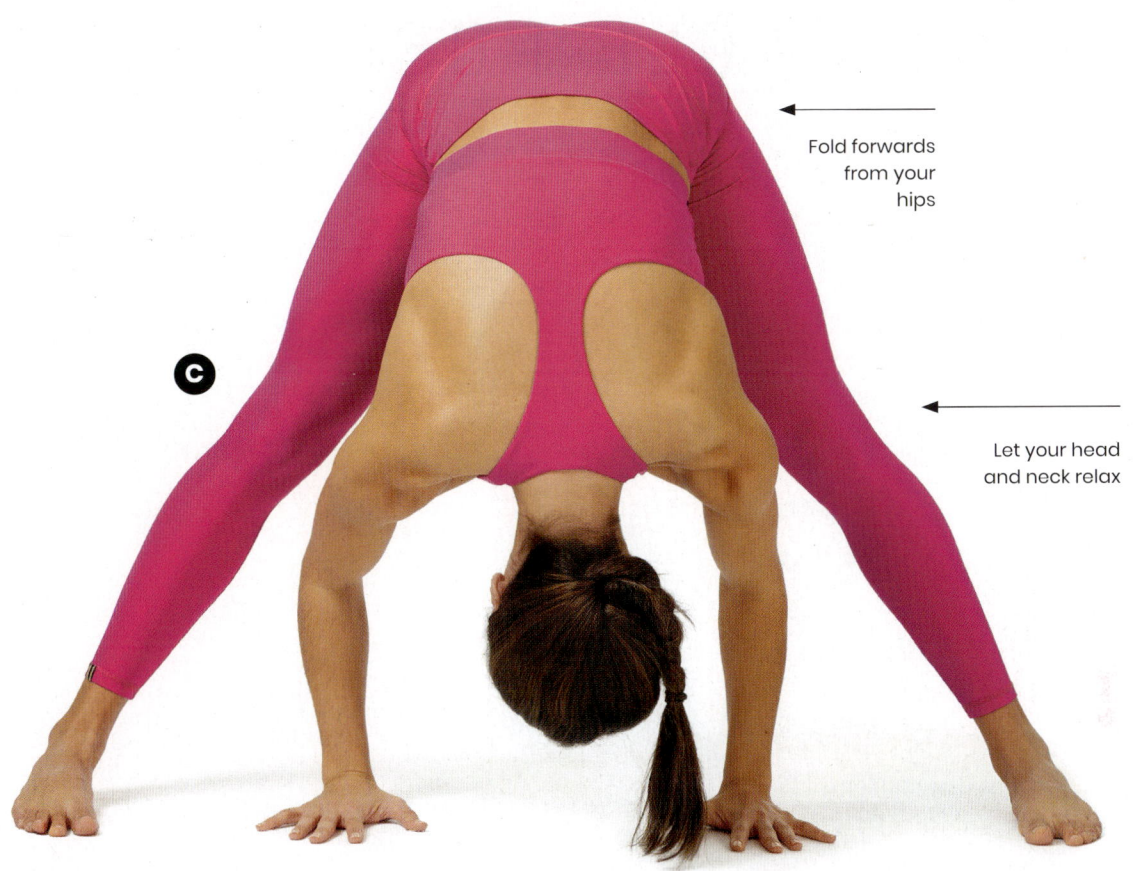

Fold forwards from your hips

Let your head and neck relax

VARIATION

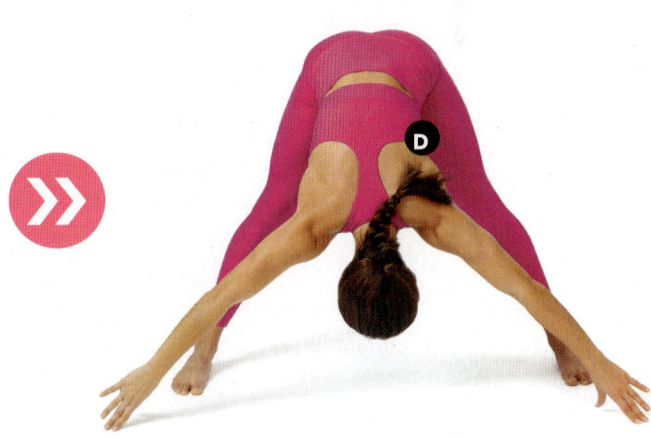

Benefits

+ Calms your mind
+ Stretches your back and hamstrings
+ Strengthens your legs
+ Relieves backache

Stretch it out
For a deeper hamstring stretch, start in Wide-legged standing forward bend (C). Take your arms out to each ankle or beyond, or a hands-length in front of your feet, and on each exhale, let your torso sink lower, feeling a gentle stretch in the back of your legs (D).

EAGLE POSE
Garudasana

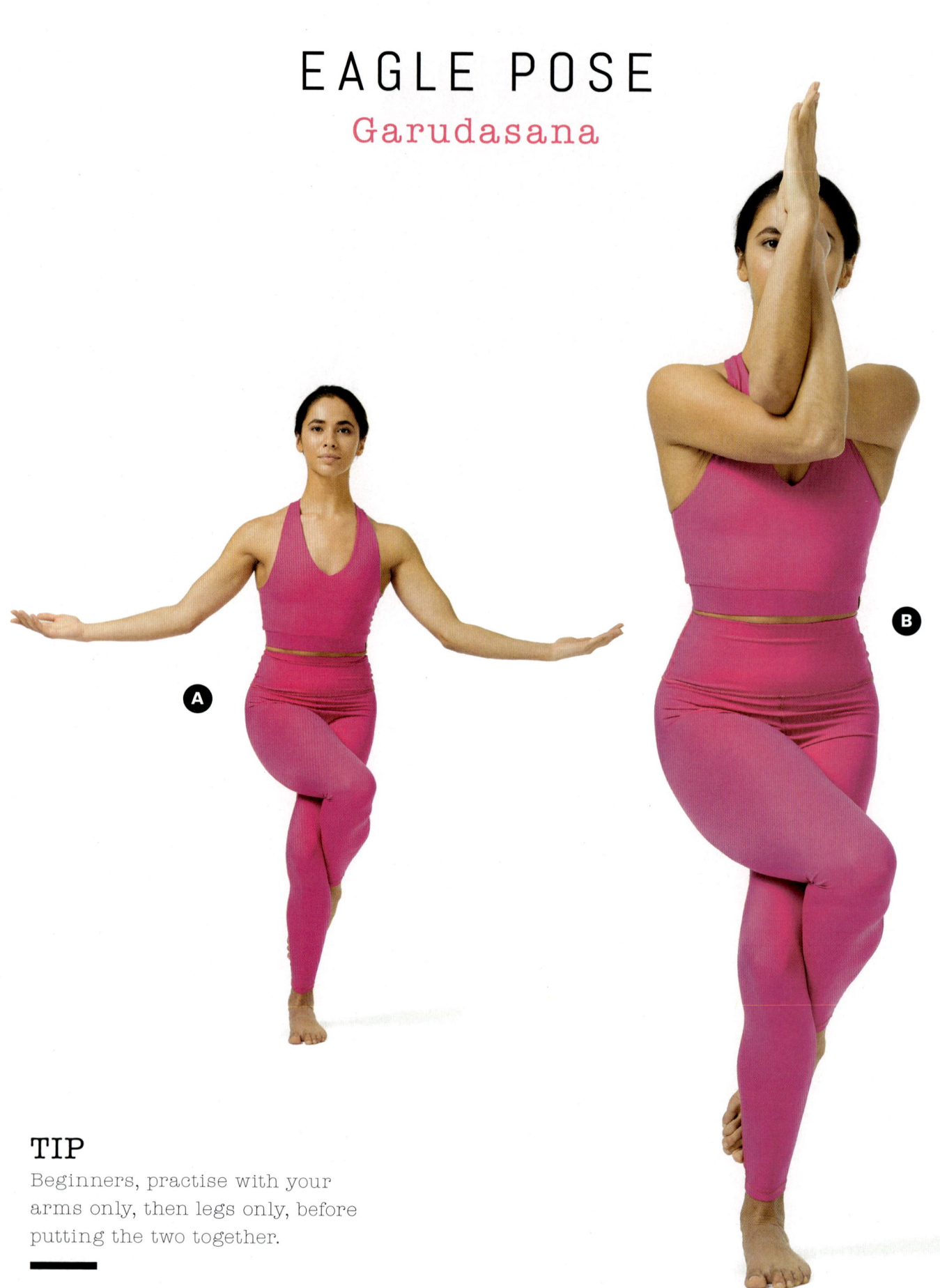

TIP
Beginners, practise with your arms only, then legs only, before putting the two together.

/ Standing poses

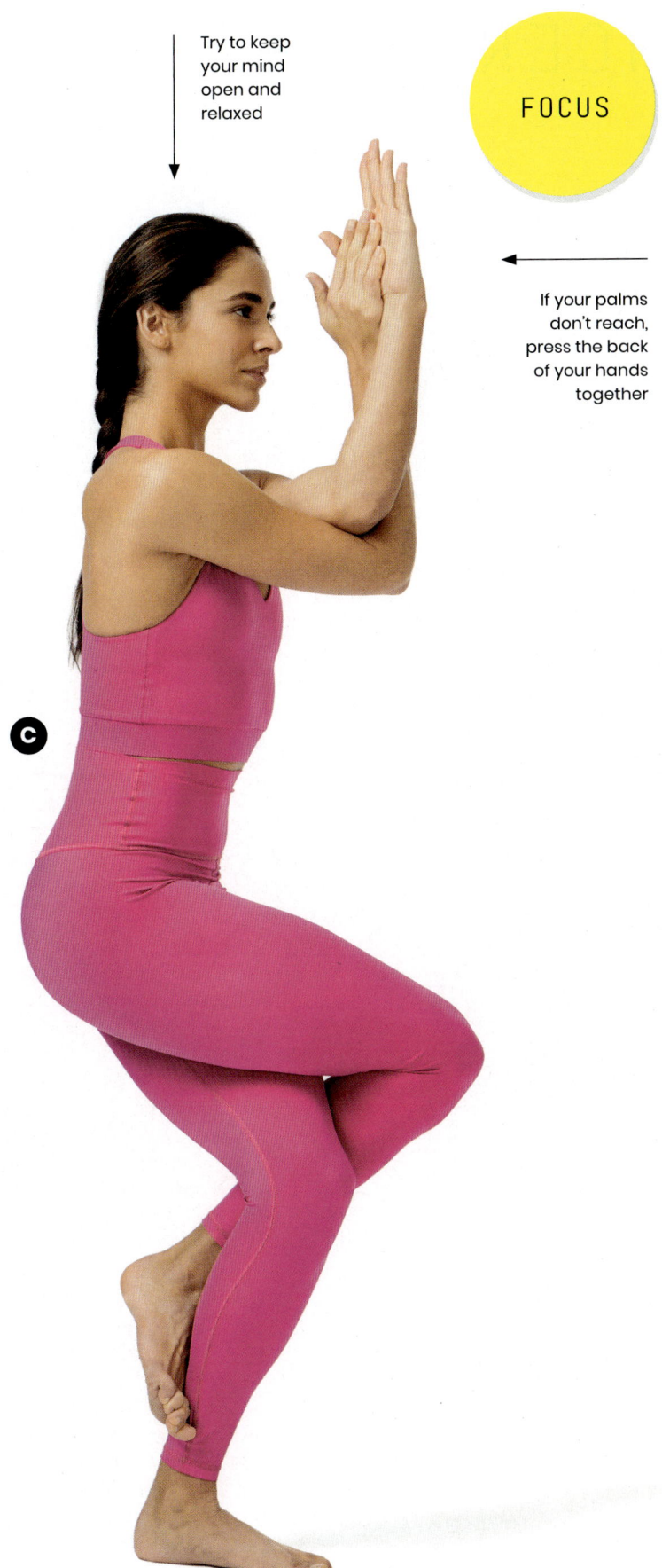

Try to keep your mind open and relaxed

FOCUS

If your palms don't reach, press the back of your hands together

■ Start in Mountain pose (p40). Spread your toes wide, root into the floor through your big and little toes, lift your arches and let your weight sink into your feet.
■ When you feel balanced, shift your weight onto your left foot, bend your left knee and place your right thigh over your left, then wrap your right shin behind your left calf, hooking your toes right round. Gaze on a fixed point ahead to aid your balance.
■ Gently inhale and float your arms out to your sides at shoulder height, palms facing up (A).
■ Exhale and cross your arms in front of you, left elbow on top of right, then intertwine your forearms to bring your palms together with your thumbs facing you and fingertips pointing up.
■ Keep your forearms vertical, draw your shoulder blades down your spine and raise your elbows to open the space between your shoulder blades (B).
■ Breathe deeply into your belly to help you stay balanced.
■ Stay in the pose for five deep breaths, then exhale and untwist your body.
■ Rest in Mountain pose, then repeat on the other side.

Benefits

+ Improves your balance
+ Aids your concentration
+ Boosts your confidence
+ Strengthens your legs

DANCER POSE
Natarajasana

EMPOWERING

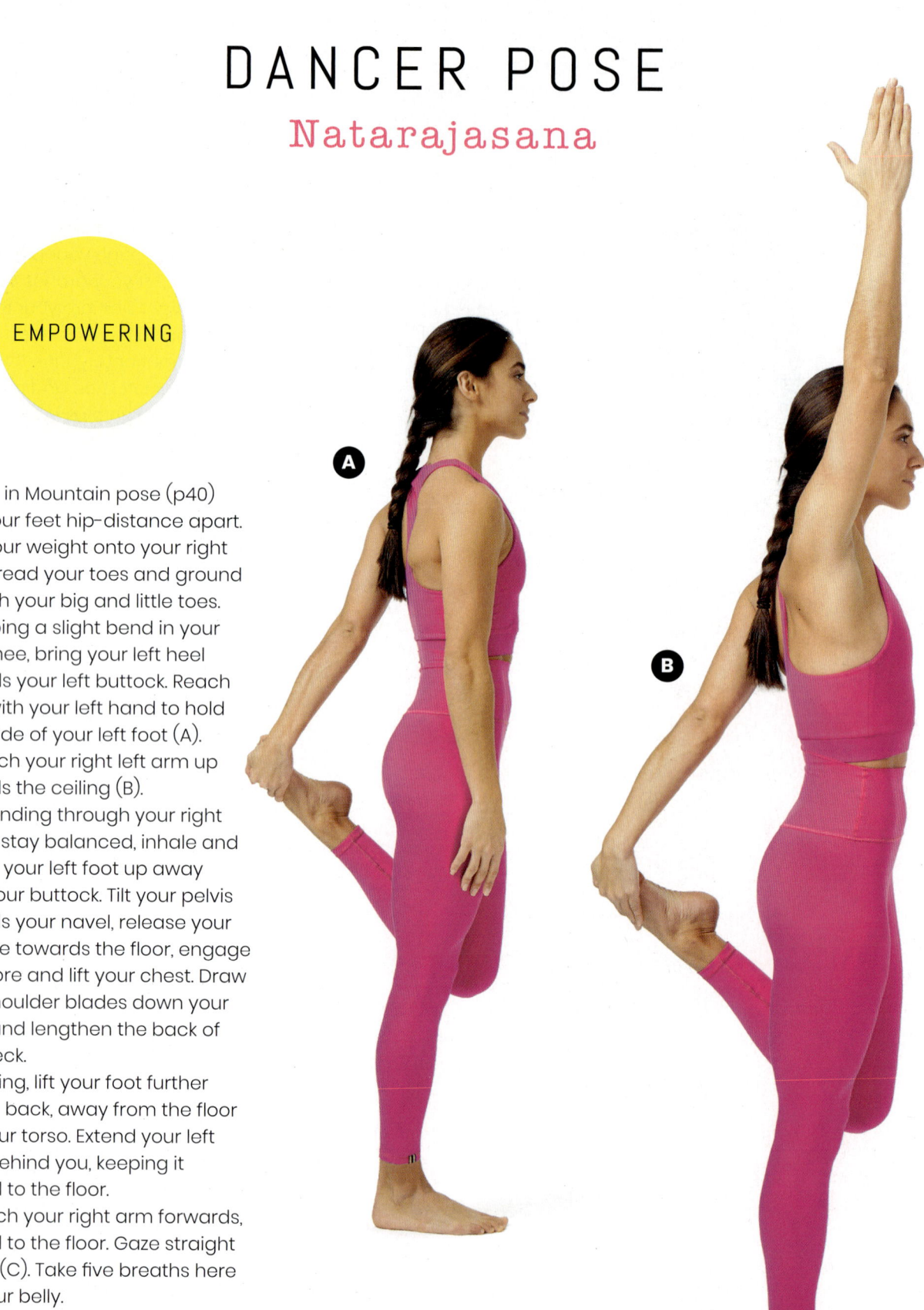

■ Start in Mountain pose (p40) with your feet hip-distance apart. Shift your weight onto your right leg. Spread your toes and ground through your big and little toes.
■ Keeping a slight bend in your right knee, bring your left heel towards your left buttock. Reach back with your left hand to hold the inside of your left foot (A).
■ Stretch your right left arm up towards the ceiling (B).
■ Grounding through your right foot to stay balanced, inhale and extend your left foot up away from your buttock. Tilt your pelvis towards your navel, release your tailbone towards the floor, engage your core and lift your chest. Draw your shoulder blades down your spine and lengthen the back of your neck.
■ Inhaling, lift your foot further up and back, away from the floor and your torso. Extend your left thigh behind you, keeping it parallel to the floor.
■ Stretch your right arm forwards, parallel to the floor. Gaze straight ahead (C). Take five breaths here into your belly.
■ To come out of the pose, exhale and release your left foot back down to the floor.
■ Repeat on the other side.

/ Standing poses

TIP
Avoid this pose if you have acute back or shoulder problems.

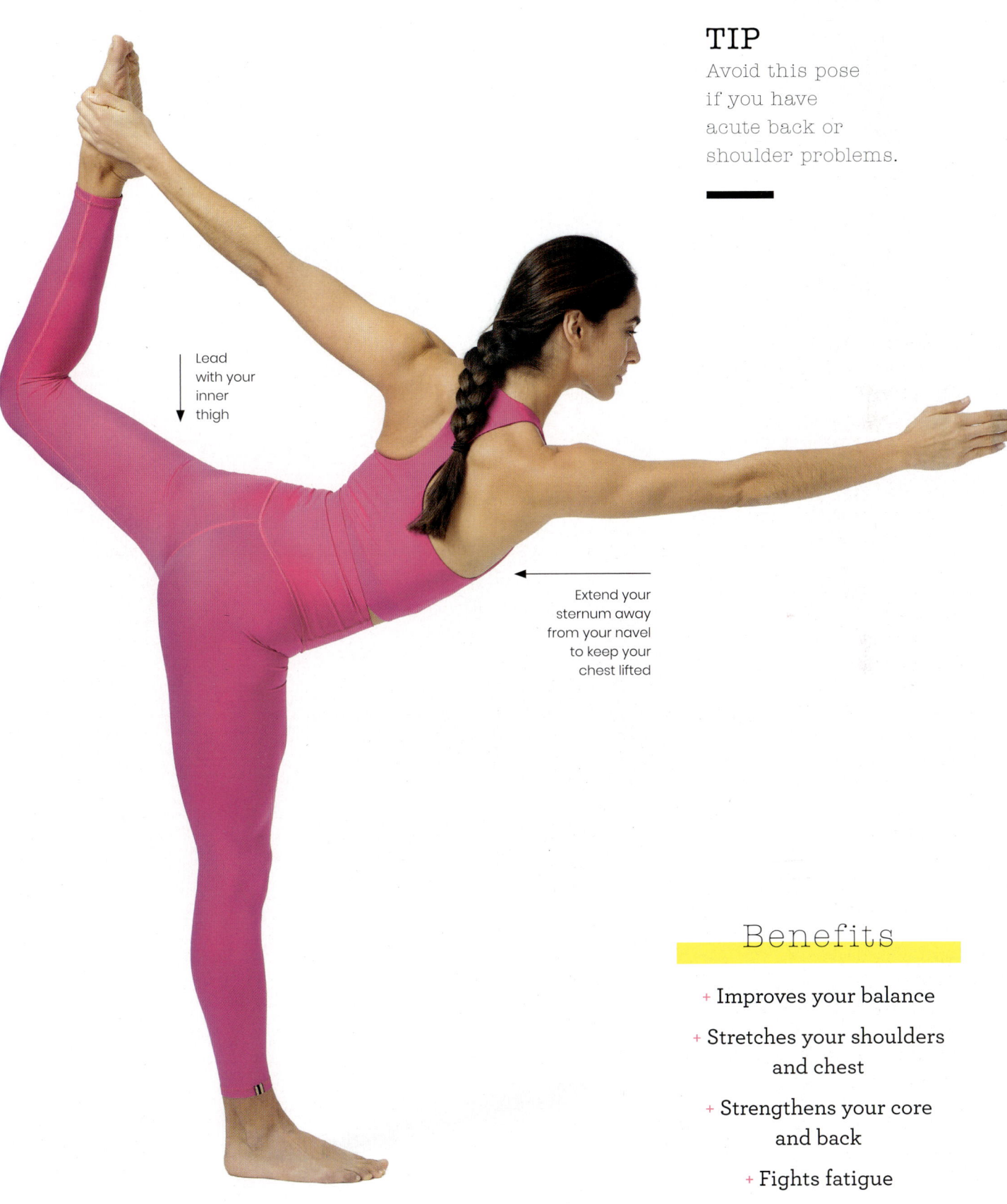

Lead with your inner thigh

Extend your sternum away from your navel to keep your chest lifted

Benefits

+ Improves your balance
+ Stretches your shoulders and chest
+ Strengthens your core and back
+ Fights fatigue

GARLAND POSE
Malasana

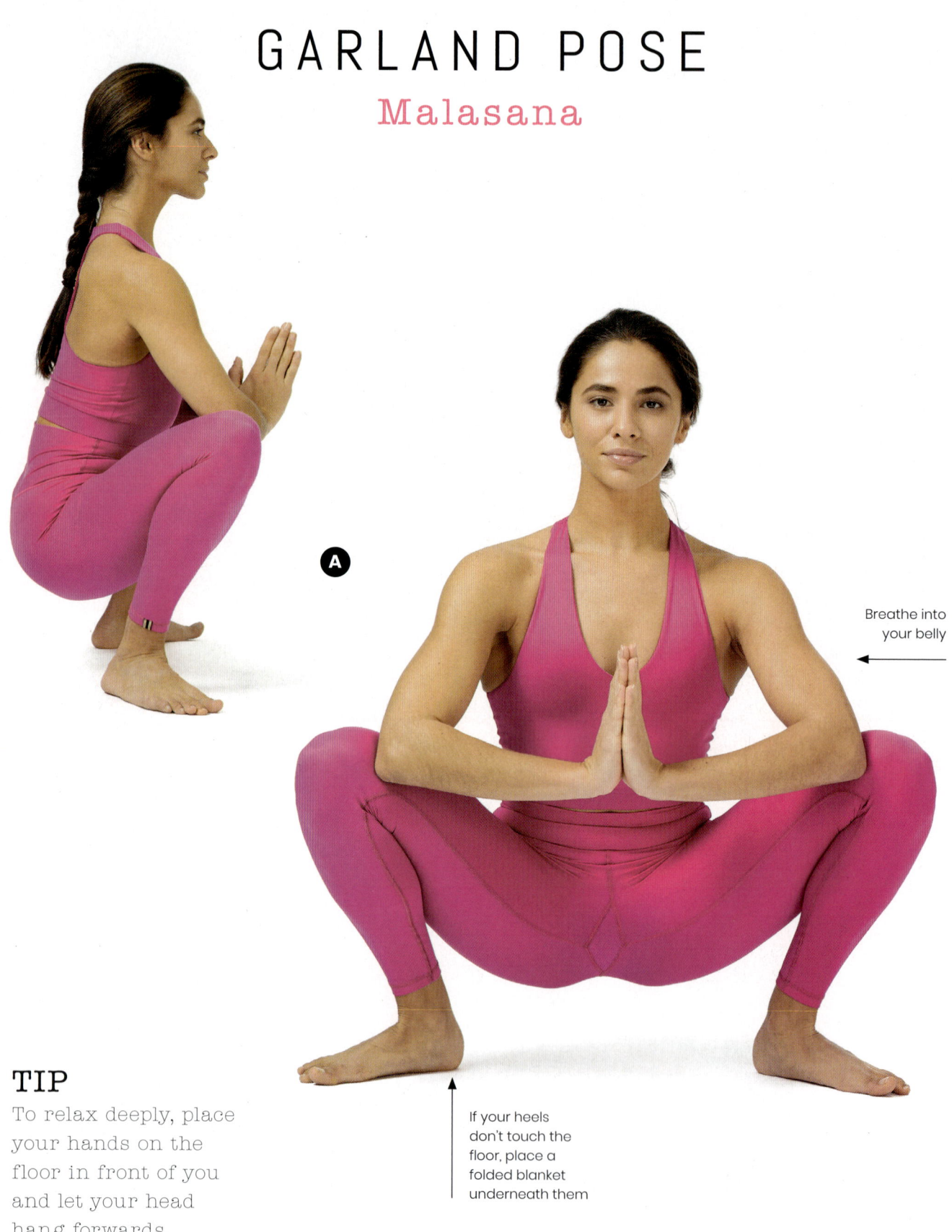

A

Breathe into your belly

If your heels don't touch the floor, place a folded blanket underneath them

TIP
To relax deeply, place your hands on the floor in front of you and let your head hang forwards.

/ Standing poses

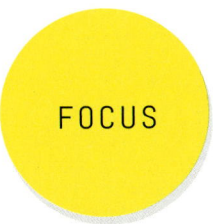

FOCUS

- Begin in Mountain pose (p40), then step your feet wider than hip-width apart.
- Exhale and lower into a deep squat, taking your hands to the floor in front of you.
- Turn your feet out so your knees are over your toes, then lower your heels, taking your feet as far apart as needed so your heels can anchor into the ground. Place your hands in Prayer position and let your tailbone release down towards the mat.
- Rooting through your feet, press your palms together and push your upper arms into your inner thighs, your thighs into your arms. This helps you lift out of your pelvis and lengthen your spine.
- Relax your shoulder blades down your back and let your chest open (A).
- Stay in the pose for five to 10 deep breaths.
- When you're ready to exit the pose, release your hands and rest in a sitting position for a few moments.

VARIATION

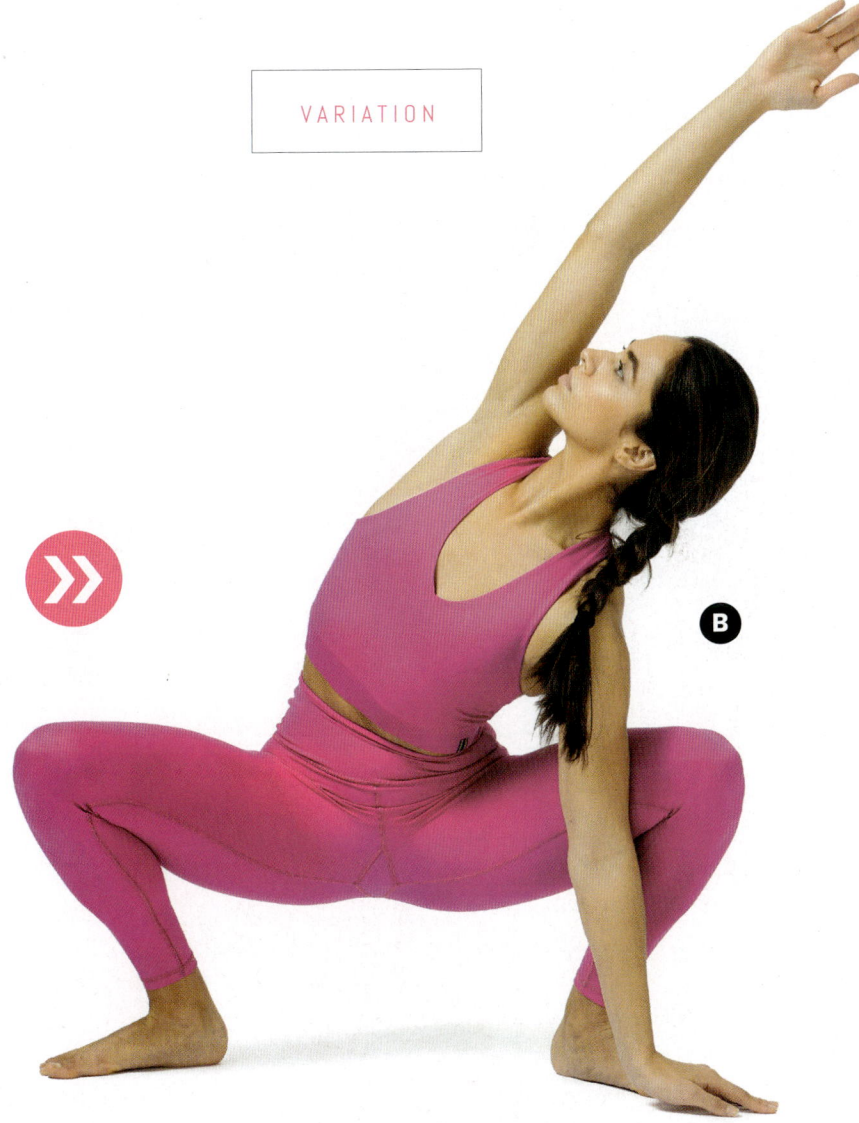

Stretch it out
- To open your hips and stretch your chest and shoulders, try Revolved squat pose. From Garland (A), place your left arm in front of your left foot then inhale and raise your right arm up to the sky. If it feels comfortable, gaze up to your right hand and reach through to your finger tips (B). Exhale and lower your right hand to the floor then continue on the other side. Repeat several times.

Benefits

+ Eases a stiff back
+ Loosens your hips
+ Stimulates digestion
+ Boosts focus

DOWNWARD-FACING DOG
Adho mukha svanasana

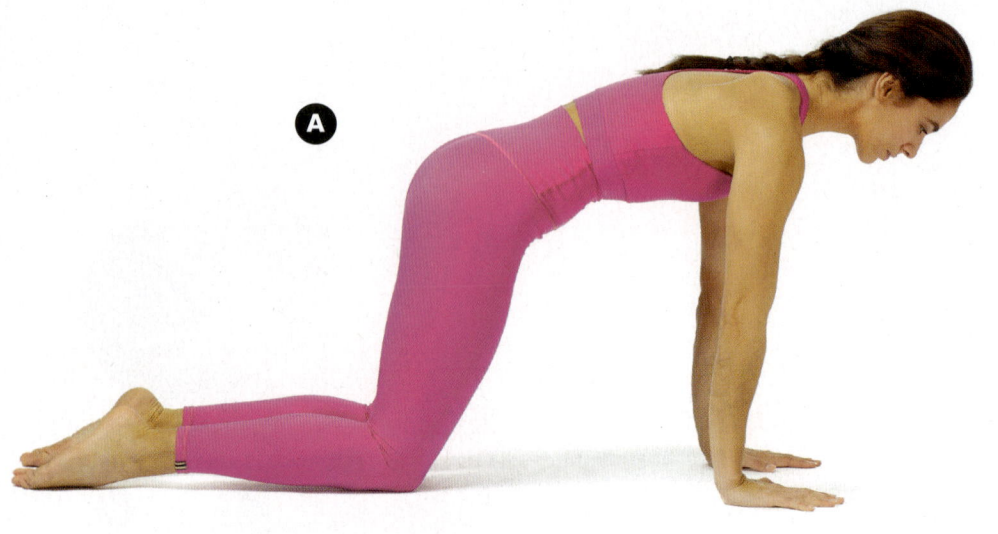

A

TIP
If your heels don't touch the floor, keep your knees slightly bent and lengthen your spine.

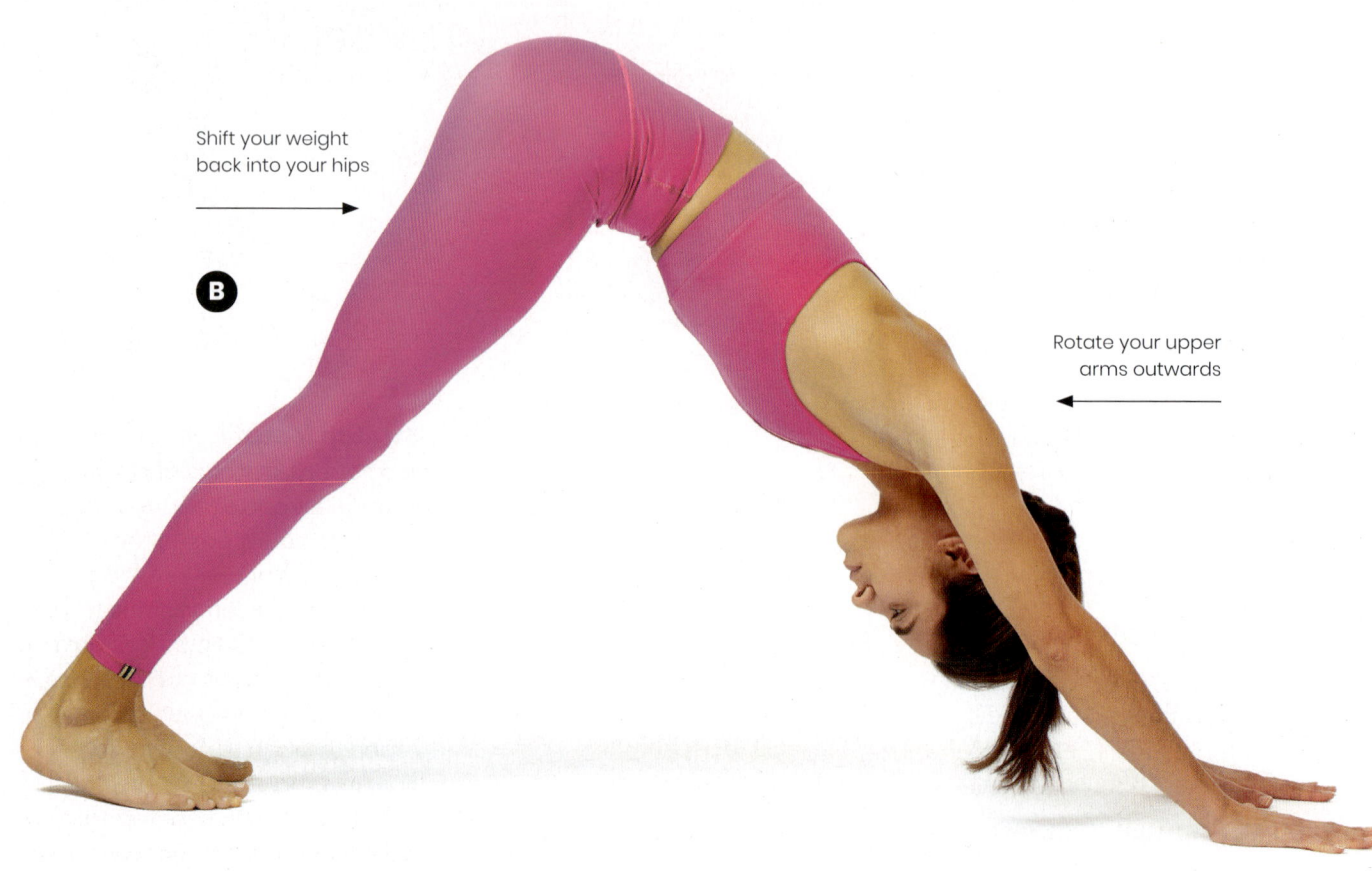

Shift your weight back into your hips →

B

← Rotate your upper arms outwards

/ Standing poses

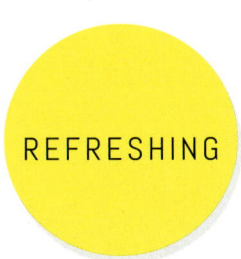

REFRESHING

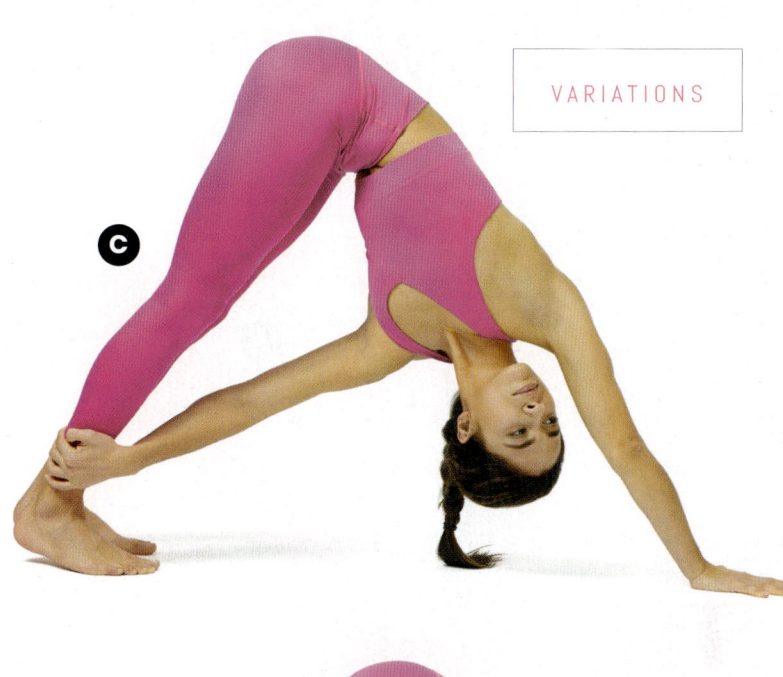

VARIATIONS

- Start on all-fours with your knees beneath your hips (A).
- Place your hands a palm's length in front of your shoulders, shoulder-width apart and fingers spread. Root through your palms.
- Tuck your toes under, draw your navel to your spine and press through your hands as you lift your hips back and up to come into an upside-down V shape.
- Keeping your knees bent, press through your hands to extend your spine. Rotate your upper arms outwards and draw your shoulder blades down your spine. Lower your ribs towards your thighs and release your neck.
- Gently draw one heel and then the other towards the mat, stretching out your hamstrings in a walking motion, then lower both heels towards the mat (B).
- Keeping your weight evenly distributed through each foot, lift the inner arches of your feet.
- Take five deep breaths here.
- To come out of the pose, exhale, bring your knees back down to the floor and lower into Child's pose (p86).

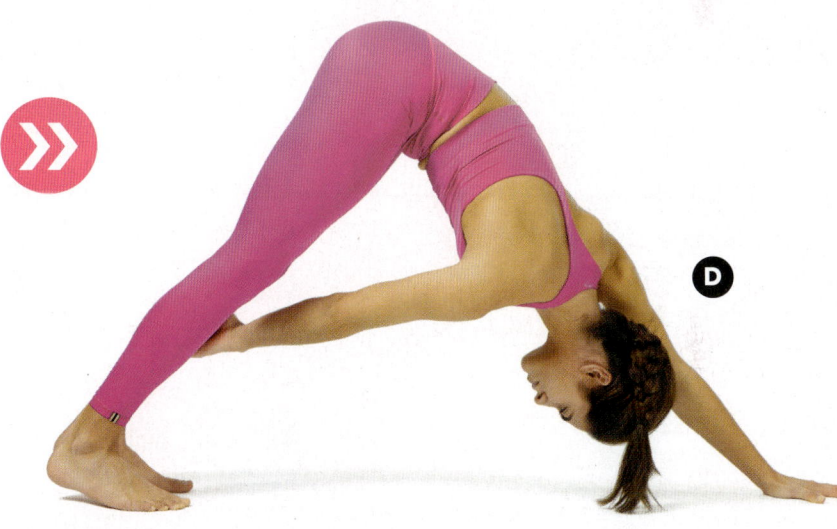

Add a twist
- To boost detoxification, aid digestion and calm stress, try Revolved downward dog pose. From Downward-facing dog (B), inhale and take your left hand down to your right ankle. Turn your head to look under your right arm and, if comfortable, gaze upwards (C). Hold for five to 10 breaths, then inhale and untwist, returning your left hand back to the mat. Repeat on the other side. If you struggle to reach your ankle, place your hand on your shin or thigh instead (D).

Benefits

+ Strengthens and tones
+ Stretches your back
+ Calms your mind
+ Revitalises your body

THREE-LIMBED DOWNWARD DOG
Eka pada adho mukha svanasana

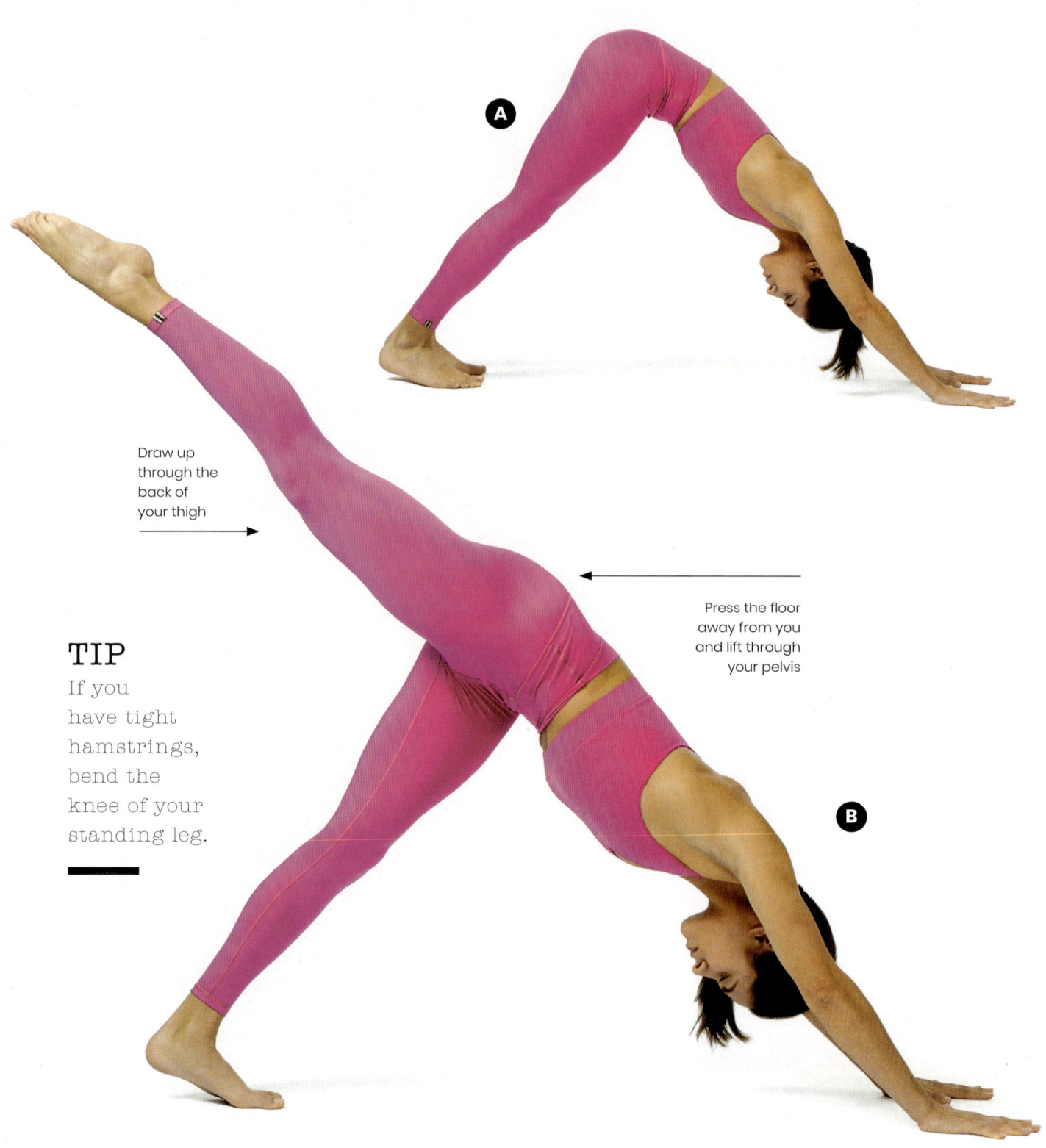

Draw up through the back of your thigh

Press the floor away from you and lift through your pelvis

TIP
If you have tight hamstrings, bend the knee of your standing leg.

Standing poses

STRENGTHEN

VARIATION

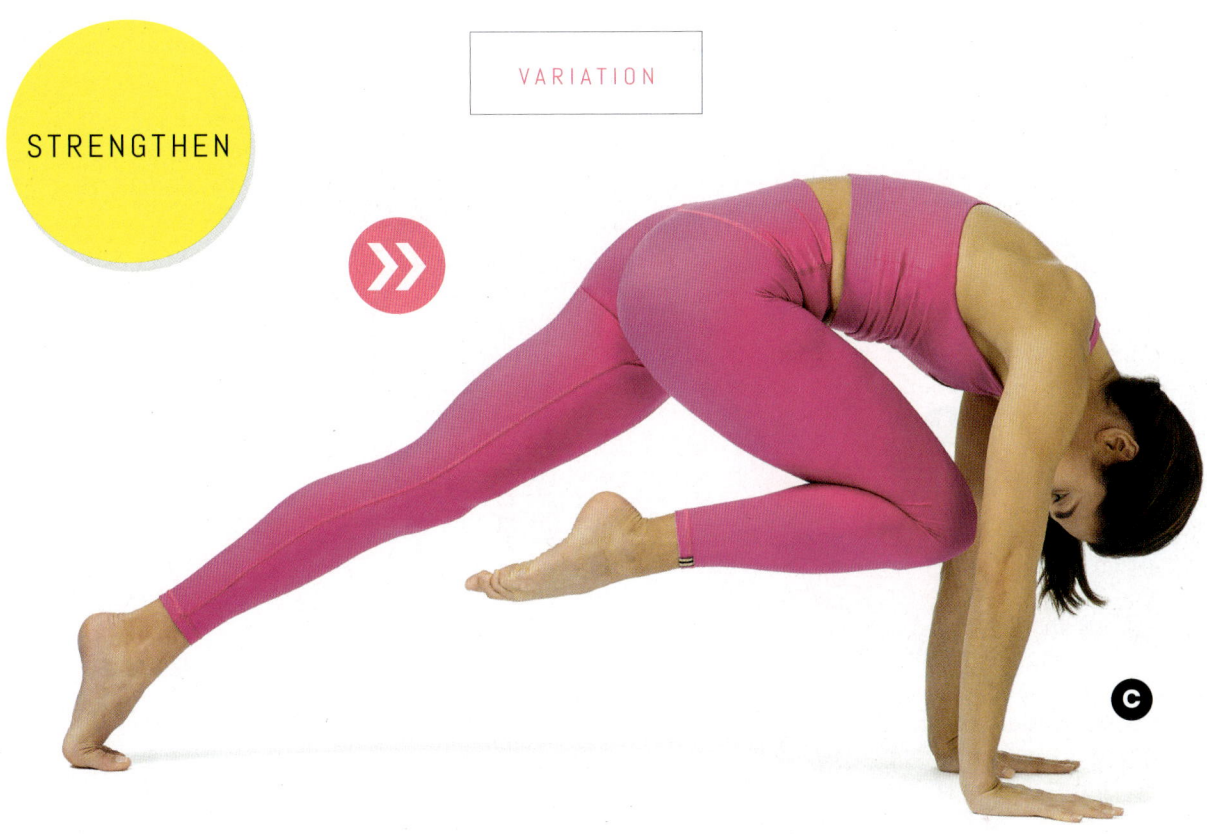

- Begin in Downward-facing dog pose (p62) and step your feet together (A).
- Root your left foot into the floor, inhale and extend your right foot back and up to the sky.
- Keep your hips square and lift from the root of your right thigh. Keep your left leg strong, press your left thigh back and lift the outer arch of your left foot.
- Square your shoulders to the top of your mat and focus on creating a straight, diagonal line from your hands to your feet.
- Root evenly through your hands and firm the outer muscles of your arms. Slids your shoulder blades down your back and lengthen both sides of your waist. Extend the crown of your head down towards the mat, gaze between your legs and stretch your right foot back and up (B).
- Stay in the pose for up to five breaths.
- Exhale and lower your leg to return to Downward-facing dog. Then repeat on the other side.

Tone your core
To challenge your balance and boost your core strength, from Three-limbed downward dog (B), exhale and shift your bodyweight forwards bringing your right knee to your nose into Knee-to-nose pose (C). Then inhale and kick your leg back into Three-limbed downward dog pose. Repeat several times, then switch sides.

Benefits

+ Improves your balance
+ Tones your legs
+ Strengthens your arms
+ Stretches your hamstrings and hips

65

PLANK
Kumbhakasana

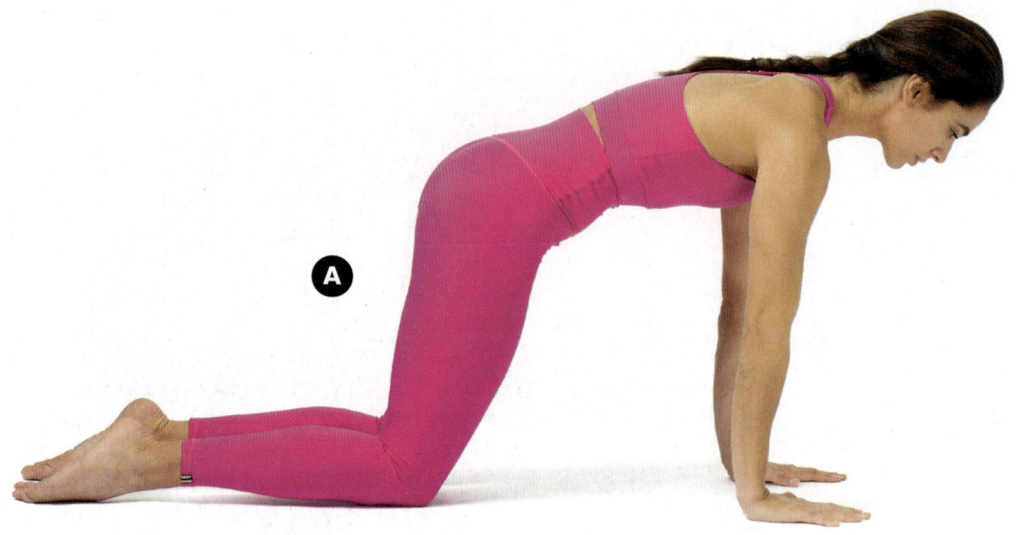

TIP
To finish, try lowering your knees to the floor and resting in Child's pose (p86).

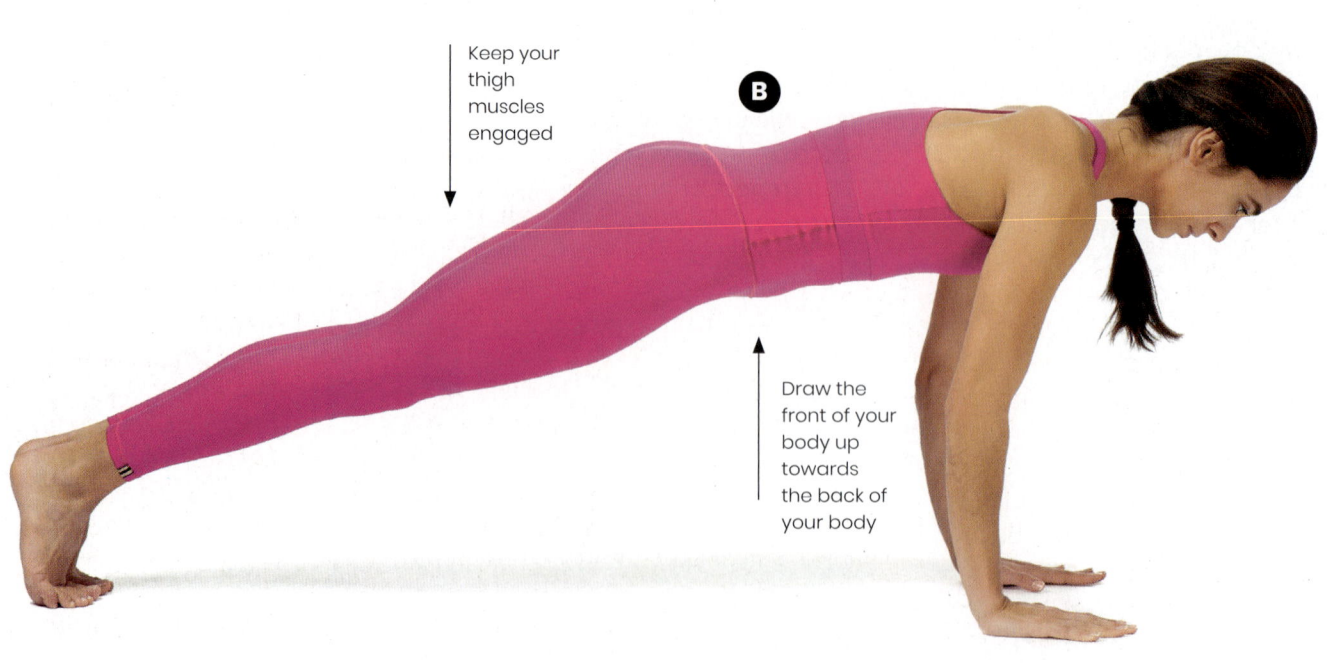

Keep your thigh muscles engaged

Draw the front of your body up towards the back of your body

/ Standing poses

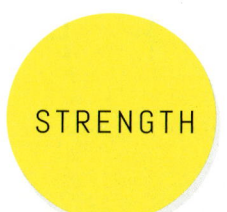

STRENGTH

- Start on all-fours with your hands under your shoulders, shoulder-width apart (A).
- Spread your fingers and root through the base of your thumbs and index fingers. Straighten your elbows but don't lock them.
- Step your feet back, resting on the balls of your feet, and straighten your legs to create a diagonal line from your heels to your crown. Tuck in your chin to keep your neck long.
- Reach your heels to the back of the room, and extend though to the crown of your head.
- Draw your navel to your spine and spread your shoulder blades (B).
- Breathe evenly for five to 10 breaths, then exhale and lower yourself gently.

VARIATION

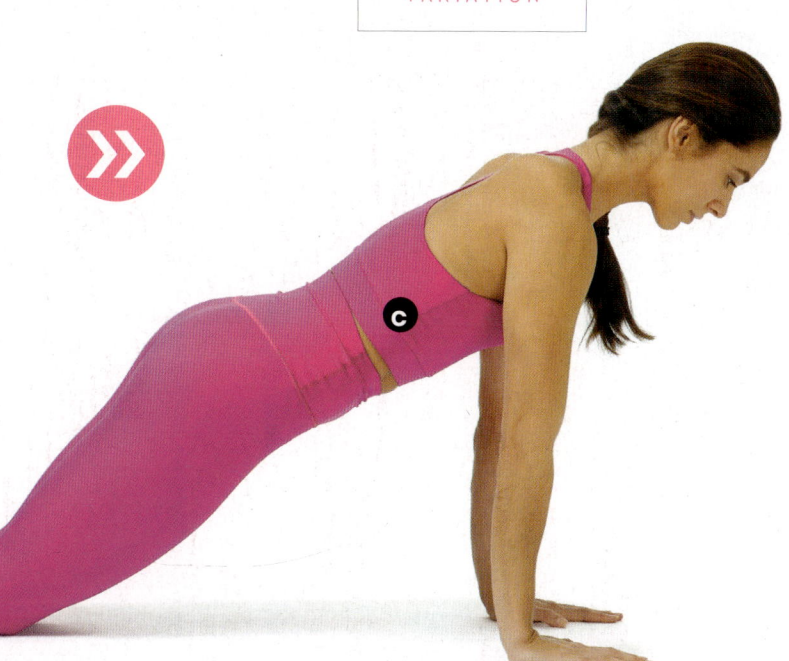

Benefits

+ Strengthens and tones your core

+ Tones your glutes

+ Strengthens your arms

+ Builds stamina

Make it easier
- If you're a beginner, you can start with Half plank. Go onto all-fours and follow the instructions for Plank but rest your knees on the floor. Ensure your hands are beneath your shoulders. Keep a straight, diagonal line from your knees to your head (C). As you build up your strength, you can progress to full Plank (B).

67

FOUR-LIMBED STAFF POSE
Chataranga dandasana

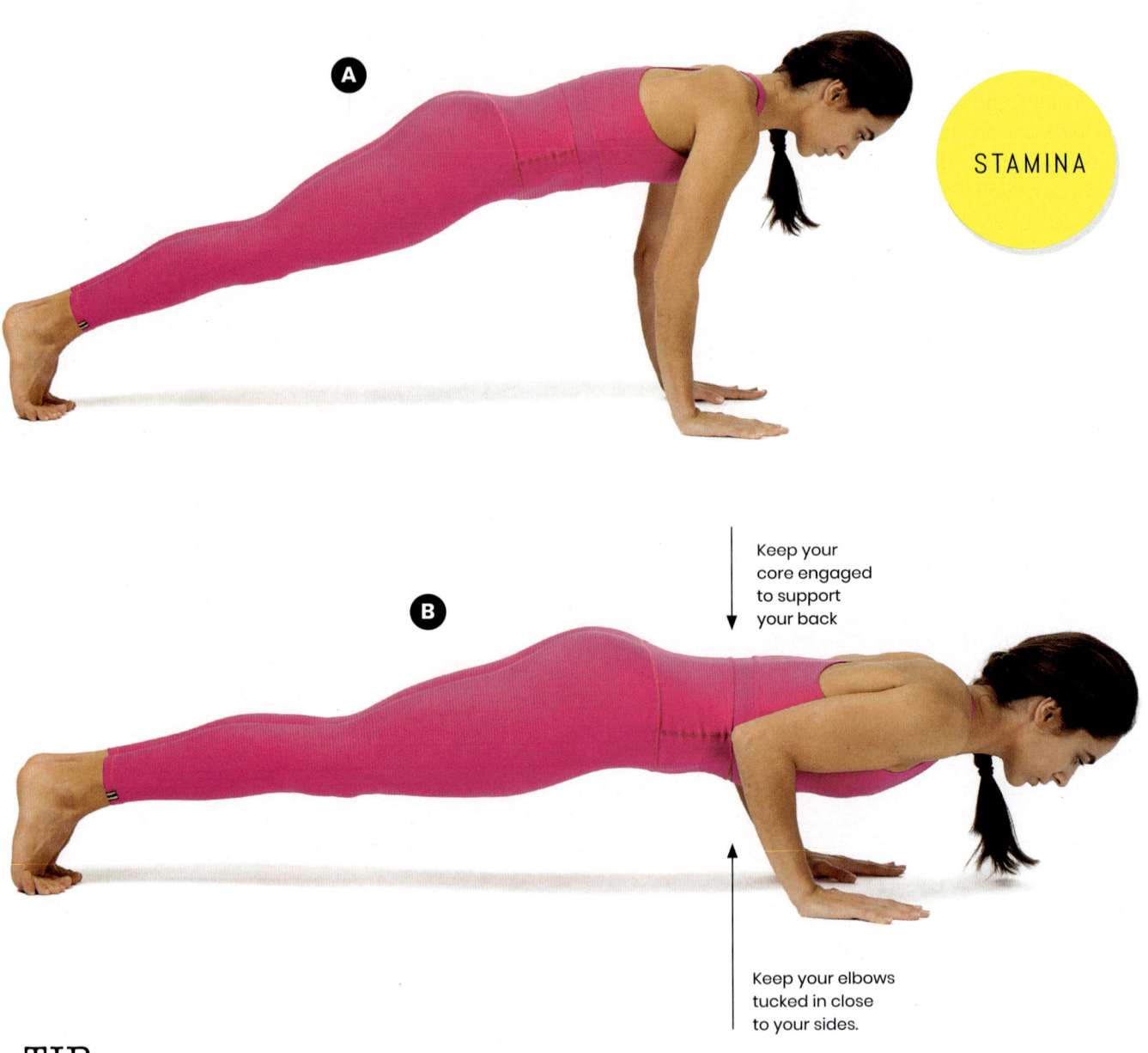

A

STAMINA

B

Keep your core engaged to support your back

Keep your elbows tucked in close to your sides.

TIP
To make it easier, from Plank (A), lower your knees to the floor before lowering your chest.

Standing poses

- Start on all-fours with your hands shoulder-width apart, directly under your shoulders.
- Step your feet back, resting on the balls of your feet and straighten your legs into Plank position (A).
- Create a diagonal line from your heels to your crown. Tuck in your chin to keep the back of your neck long.
- Take your body forwards so your shoulders are beyond your hands. Exhale and lower your body, so your upper arms are horizontal while your forearms remain vertical.
- Engage your legs and reach backwards with your heels. Draw your navel into your spine, broaden your shoulder blades and press the base of your index fingers into the floor (B).
- Breathe into your belly and stay in the pose for five to 10 breaths.
- When you're ready to come out of the pose, lower slowly onto your stomach or exhale and push back up to straight arms, then lower onto your knees to rest in Child's pose (p86).

Benefits

+ Sculpts your arms
+ Strengthens your arms and shoulders
+ Tones your abdominals
+ Builds stamina

VARIATION

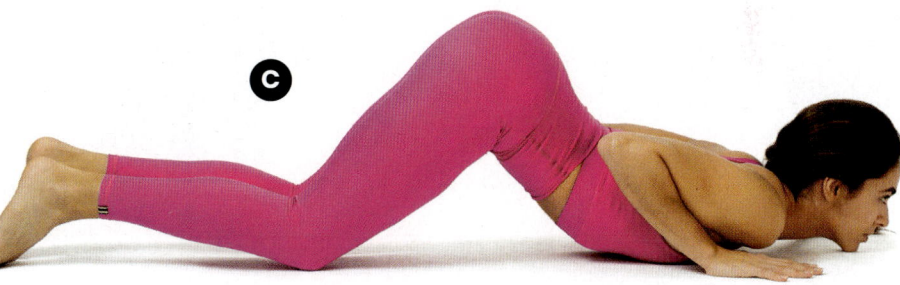

Boost your energy
- Four-limbed staff pose (B) is often included in sequences such as Sun salutation (p102). Another transition pose is Eight-limbed pose or Caterpillar, often practised before coming into Cobra (p72) to help boost your energy. From kneeling, walk your hands forwards and, exhaling, slide your torso forwards so your chest and chin are on the mat. Keep your legs together, toes tucked under, elbows tucked in. Push down on your hands and press forwards with your toes. Hold for a breath.

LIZARD POSE
Utthan pristhasana

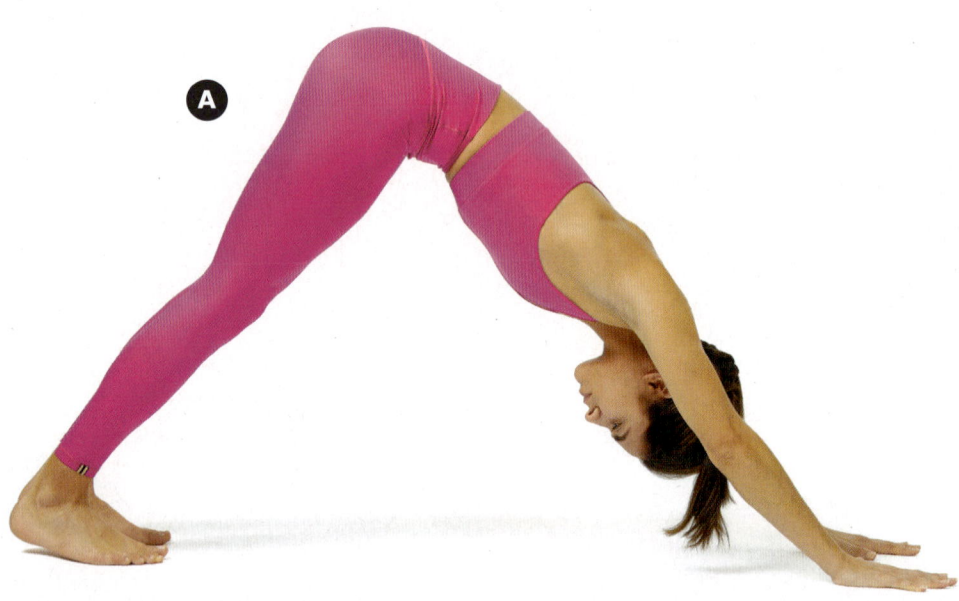

TIP
If you find this stretch uncomfortable, lower your back knee to the floor.

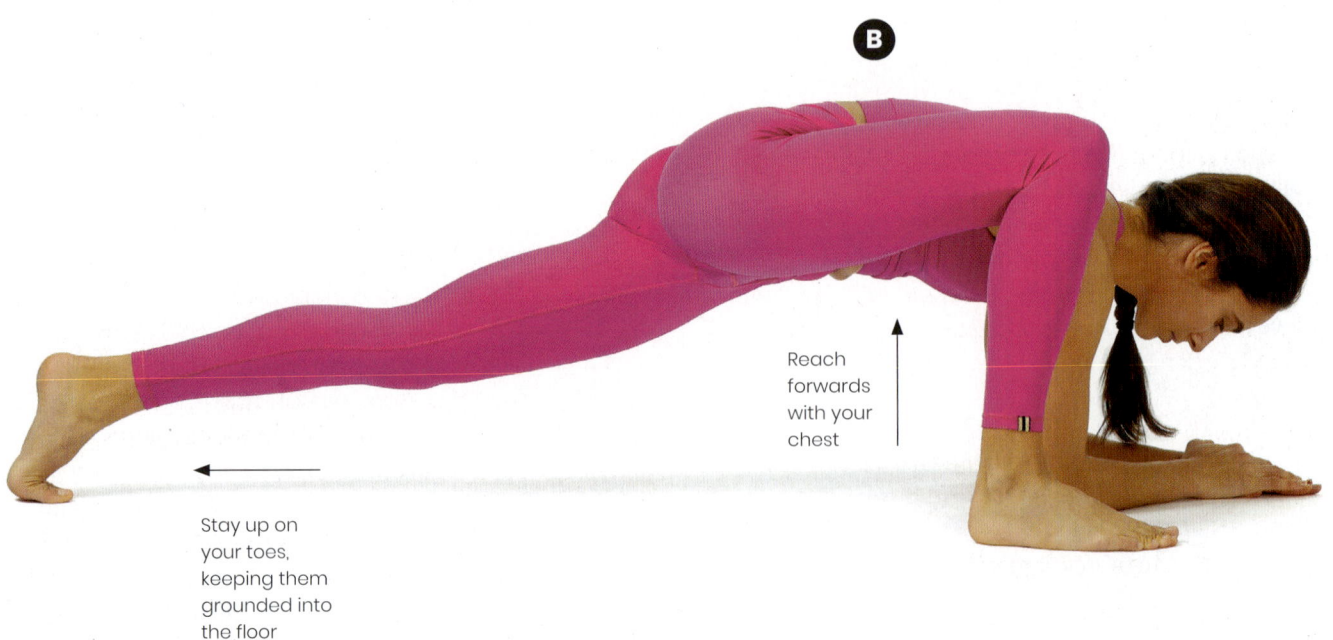

Reach forwards with your chest

Stay up on your toes, keeping them grounded into the floor

/ Standing poses

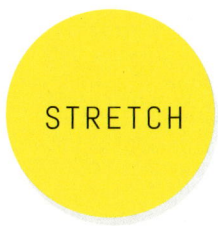

STRETCH

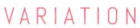

VARIATION

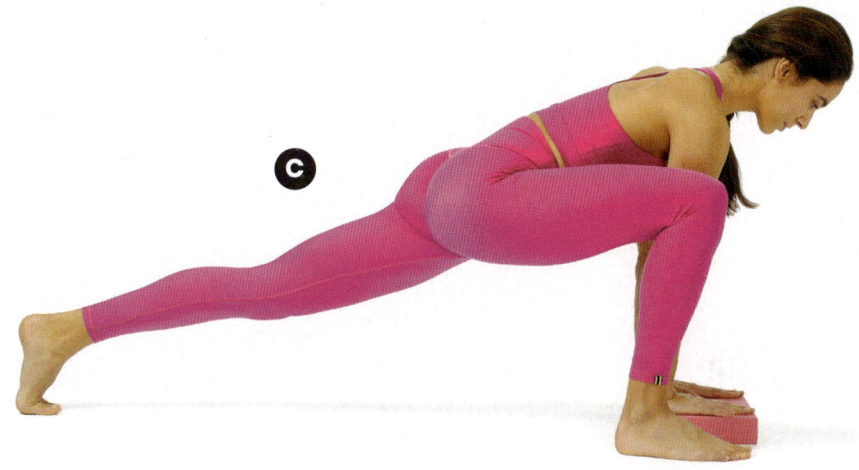

■ From Downward-facing dog (p62) (A) step your right foot forwards between your hands. Raise your right hand and shift your right foot towards the edge of your mat, then lower your hand back down so it's inside your foot.
■ Keep your right knee directly above your ankle, tuck your back toes under and ground through the base of your big and little toes.
■ Walking your hands slightly forwards, sink your hips forwards and down, draw your shoulder blades down your back. Extend your chest forwards to lengthen your spine.
■ Engage your core by gently drawing your navel to your spine.
■ If comfortable, gently rest your forearms on the floor, keeping your chin lifted.
■ Press up into the ball of your left foot, press back with your left heel and activate your inner left thigh (B).
■ Remain in the pose for five deep breaths, then press your hands into the mat and step your right leg back into Downward-facing dog. Rest here and repeat on the other side.

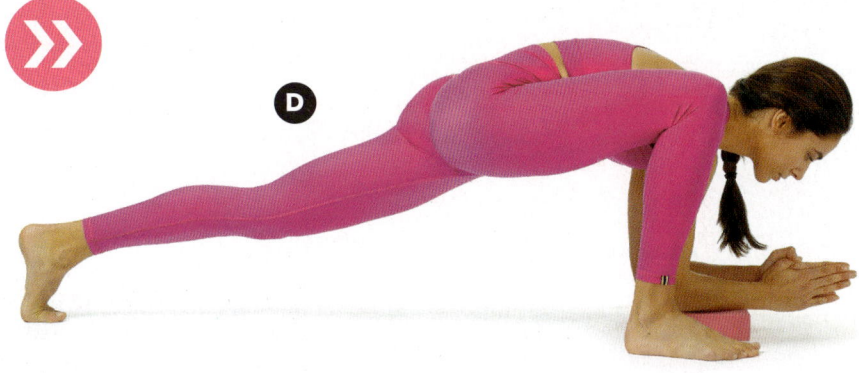

Make it easier
■ If you're a beginner or struggle to get your forearms onto the floor, try using a block to support you. Follow the instructions left, but place the block under your hands when you step forwards from Downward-facing dog (C). Stay here for a few, deep breaths or gently lower your forearms down onto the block as you come forwards into the full pose (D). As your hip flexibility improves, you'll be able to remove the block.

Benefits

+ Opens your hips
+ Stretches your hamstrings and thighs
+ Strengthens your legs
+ Reduces stress

COBRA
Bhujangasana

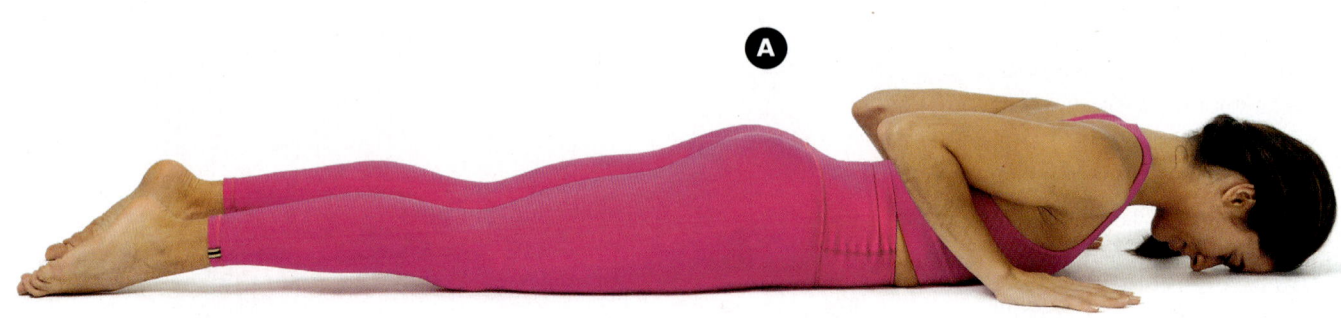

TIP
Keep a slight bend in your elbows.

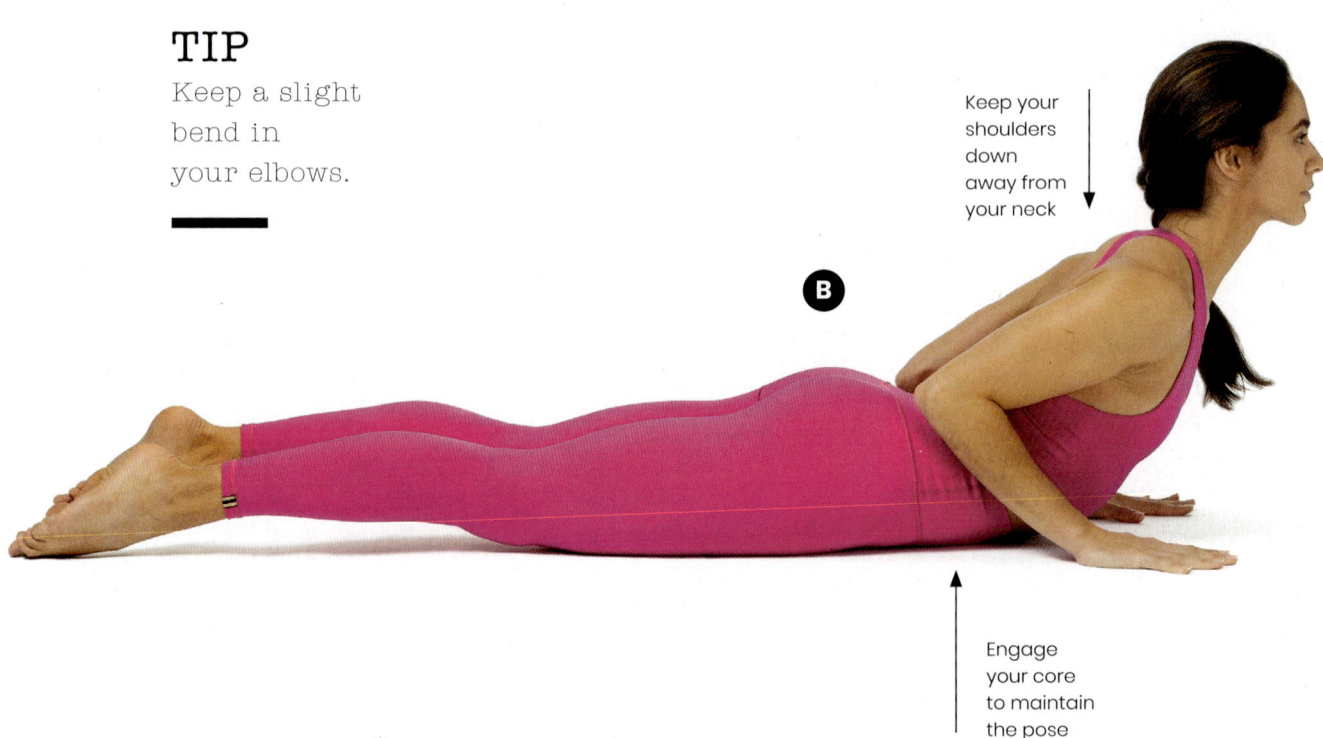

Keep your shoulders down away from your neck

Engage your core to maintain the pose

Backbend poses

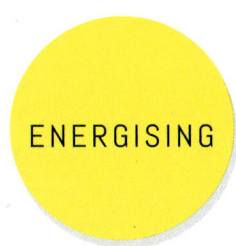

ENERGISING

- Lie on your stomach, with your legs straight and feet hip-distance apart.
- Rest your forehead on the floor and place your hands beneath your shoulders, palms facing down and fingers spread (A).
- Bring your elbows in and draw your shoulder blades back and down to create space around your neck.
- Draw your navel to your spine, root through your pubic bone and inhale, pressing through your hands to raise your head and shoulders. Exhale.
- Now inhale and lengthen through your spine, lifting your head to look forwards. Reach through the crown of your head to the ceiling (B).
- Stay in the pose for five to 10 breaths. On each exhale, draw your shoulders down.
- Exhale and slowly lower your body to the floor. Rest your head on one side for a moment or two.

Benefits

+ Revives your body and mind
+ Improves your posture
+ Strengthens your back
+ Stretches your chest and abdomen

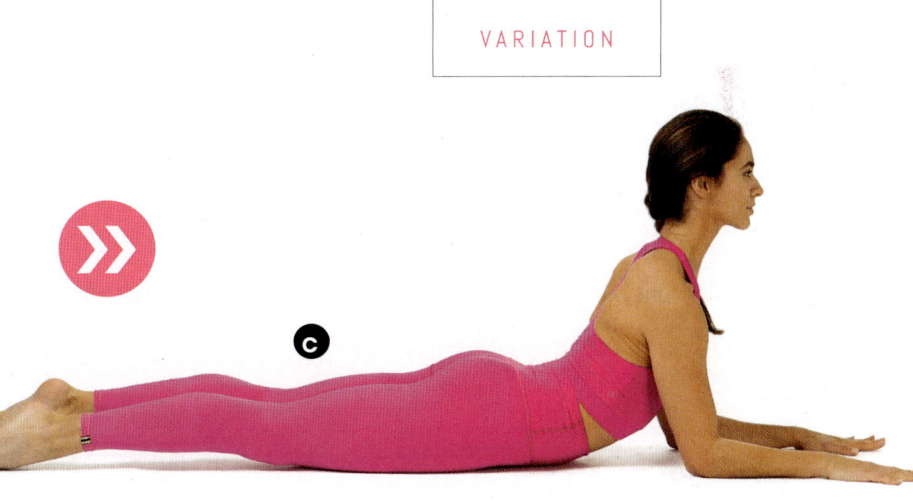

VARIATION

Make it easier
For a gentler backbend, try Sphinx pose. Begin in the start pose (A), with your thighs inwardly rotated and reaching through your toes. Inhale and place your elbows under your shoulders, forearms on the floor. Inhale and lift the top of your torso and head up from the floor into a slight backbend. Draw your navel into your spine to support you (C). Stay in the pose for several breaths, then exhale and gently lower your torso back to the floor. Rest your head on one side for a moment or two.

UPWARD-FACING DOG POSE
Urdhva mukha svanasana

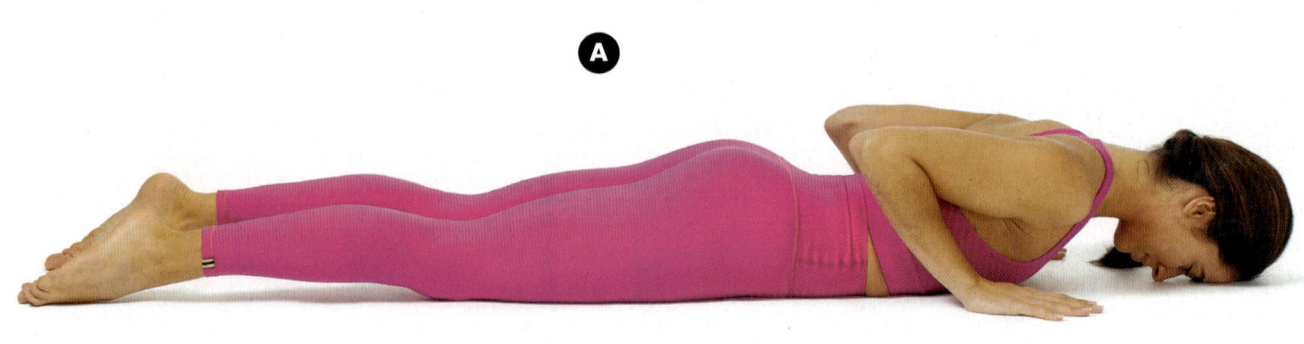

TONING

- Begin lying face down on the floor with your feet facing downwards, arms by your sides.
- Bend your elbows and bring your palms on the floor under your shoulders (A).
- Press the tops of your feet into the floor and engage your thighs.
- Inhale, press your palms into the floor and straighten your arms, lifting your torso and legs off the floor.
- Keep your legs active by squeezing your thigh muscles together. Your weight should be resting on your feet and palms (B).
- Draw your shoulder blades back, keeping your chest lifted. Look forwards or upwards.
- Stay in the pose for one to five deep breaths.
- To come out of the pose, exhale and lower back to the floor or lift your hips up into Downward-facing dog pose (p62).

/ Backbend poses

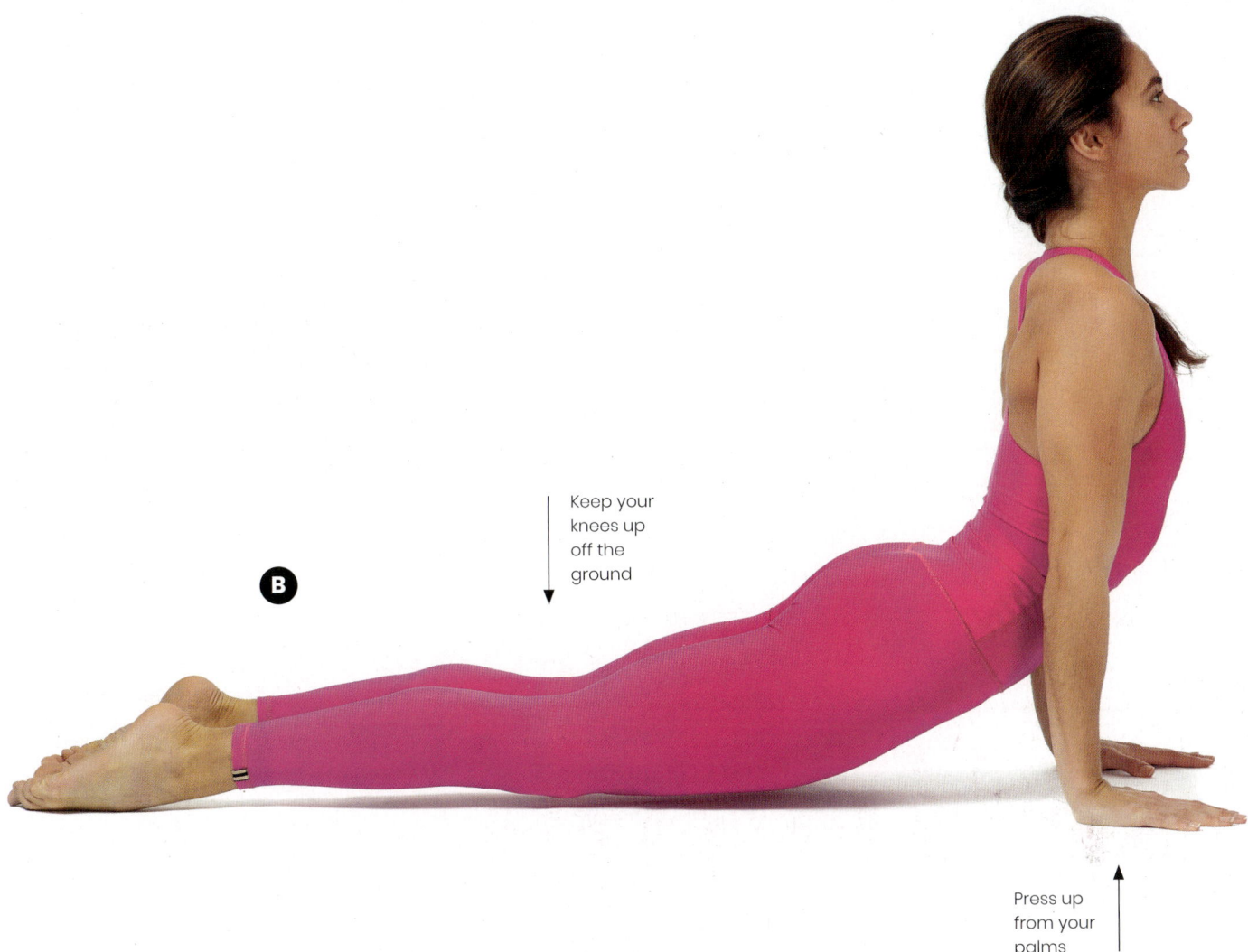

Keep your knees up off the ground

B

Press up from your palms

TIP
This pose is good for counteracting long hours sitting at a desk.

Benefits

+ Opens your chest
+ Strengthens your arms and wrists
+ Stretches your core, chest and shoulders
+ Tones your bum

LOCUST
Salabasana

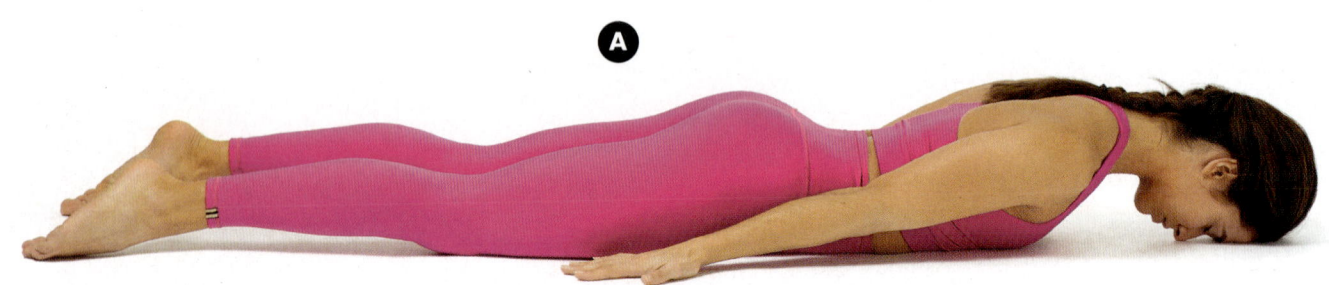

TIP
If you find this pose uncomfortable, try placing a folded blanket underneath your pelvis.

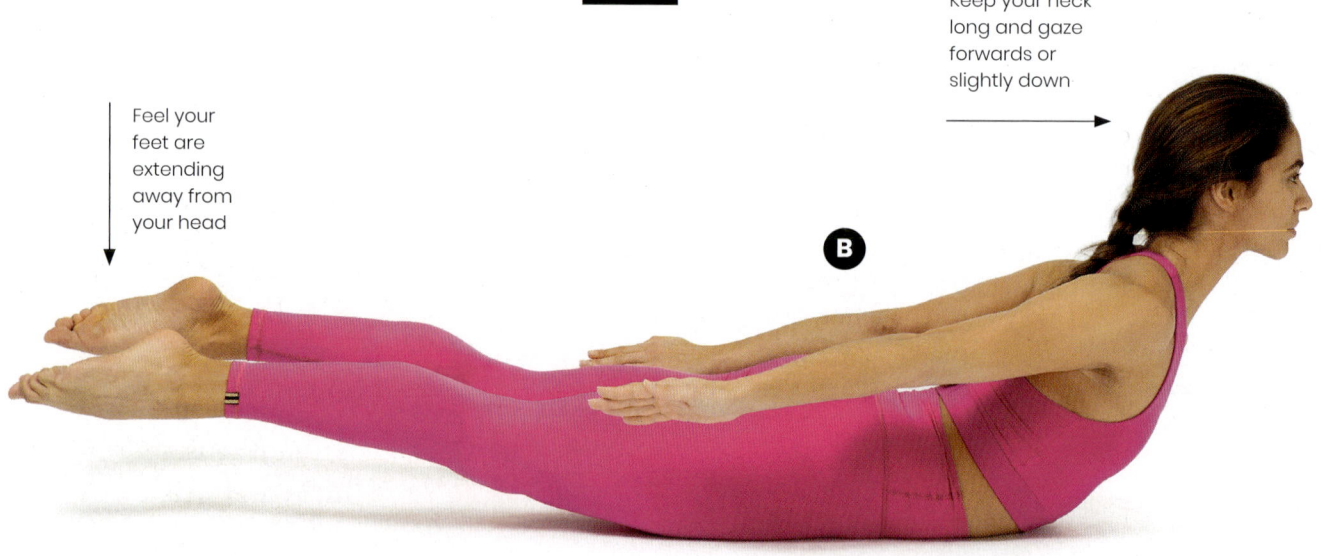

Feel your feet are extending away from your head

Keep your neck long and gaze forwards or slightly down

/ Backbend poses

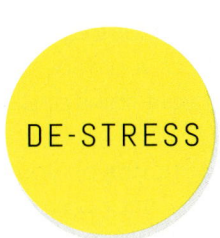

DE-STRESS

VARIATIONS

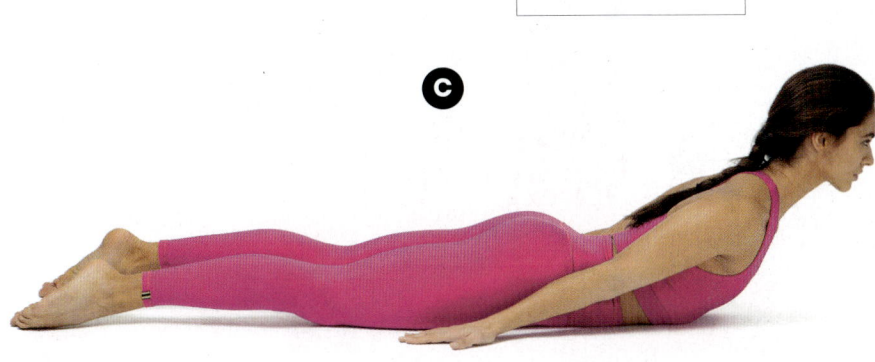

C

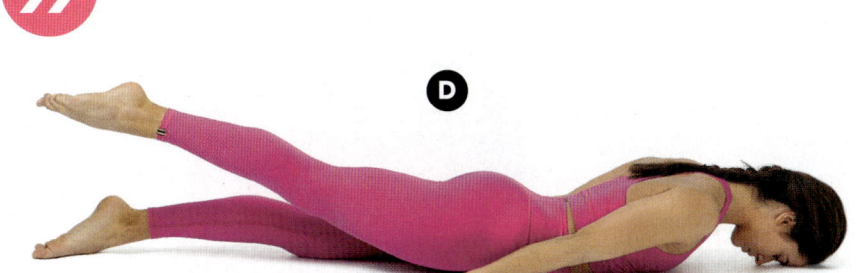

D

- Lie face down on the floor with your chin resting on the mat and your arms alongside your torso, palms facing downwards.
- Keep your big toes facing towards each other and firm your buttocks, drawing your tailbone towards your pelvis (A).
- Exhale, draw your navel to your spine and raise your head, arms, chest and legs off the floor so you're resting on your lower ribs, stomach and lower abdomen.
- Raise your arms parallel to the floor, stretching through your fingertips and pressing your shoulderblades into your back.
- Firm your buttocks and extend strongly through your legs to your pointed toes and through your fingertips. Engage your glutes, lengthen the back of your neck and gaze forwards (B).
- Remain in the pose for 30 seconds to one minute, breathing slowly and evenly.
- To come out of the pose, exhale and release your body to the floor, resting your head on your folded arms, face pointing to the side.
- Repeat two to three times.

Benefits

+ Strengthens your lower back, legs and arms
+ Opens your chest and shoulders
+ Relieves stress
+ Prepares your body for backbends

Make it easier
- If you're a beginner or find the full pose challenging, try raising just your head and chest off the floor as you inhale (C). Hold for a few breaths, then lower yourself to your mat. Or try lifting one leg at a time. From the start pose (A), engage your core, draw your pubic bone into the floor and lift your right leg up, firming it and stretching it back. Keep your neck long and gaze down to keep your spine aligned (D).

CAMEL
Ustrasana

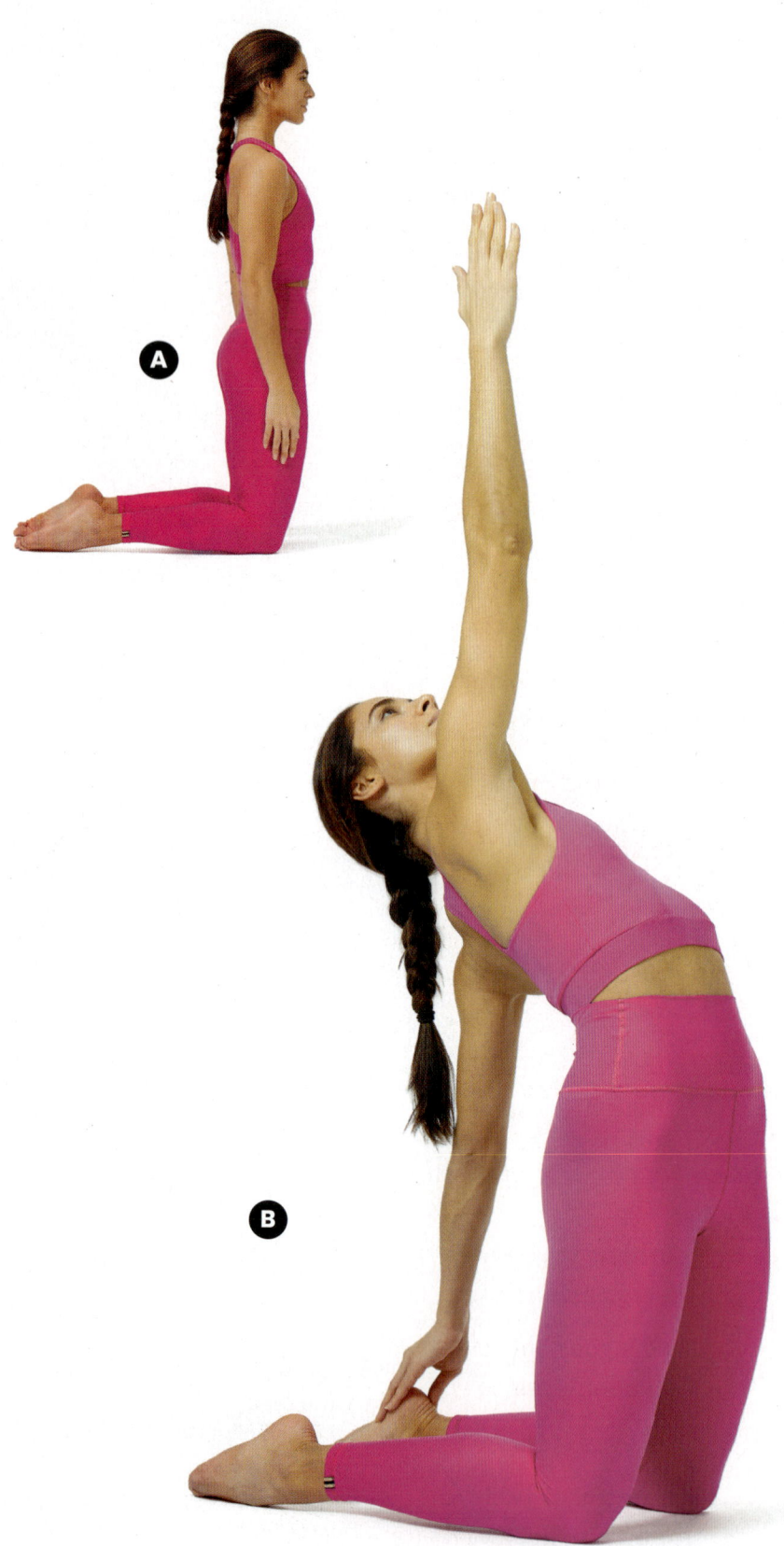

- Kneel with your thighs hip-width apart, tops of your feet flat on the floor. Root your shins and feet into the floor (A).
- Rest your hands on your lower back, base of your palms on the top of your buttocks. Draw your tailbone forwards and press the front of your thighs back. Draw your shoulders down your back.
- Keeping your tailbone firm, lean back and drop your left hand down to your left heel.
- Inhale and raise your right arm up over your head. If your neck feels comfortable, take your head back and look up to your hand (B).
- Stay here for a few breaths.
- Once you're ready to come back up, bring your hands to your hips, inhale and carefully lift your head and torso up by pushing your hips towards the floor while leading with your chest.
- Repeat on the other side.
- For the full pose, drop your right hand to your right heel and your left hand to your left heel.
- Exhale, lifting your chest and shoulders. Draw your tailbone under and your pubic bone upwards. If your neck feels comfortable, take your head back and look up (C).
- Take a few breaths here.
- To come out of the pose, bring your hands to your hips, inhale and carefully lift your head and torso up by pushing your hips towards the floor while leading with your chest.
- Rest in Child's pose (p86).

/ Backbend poses

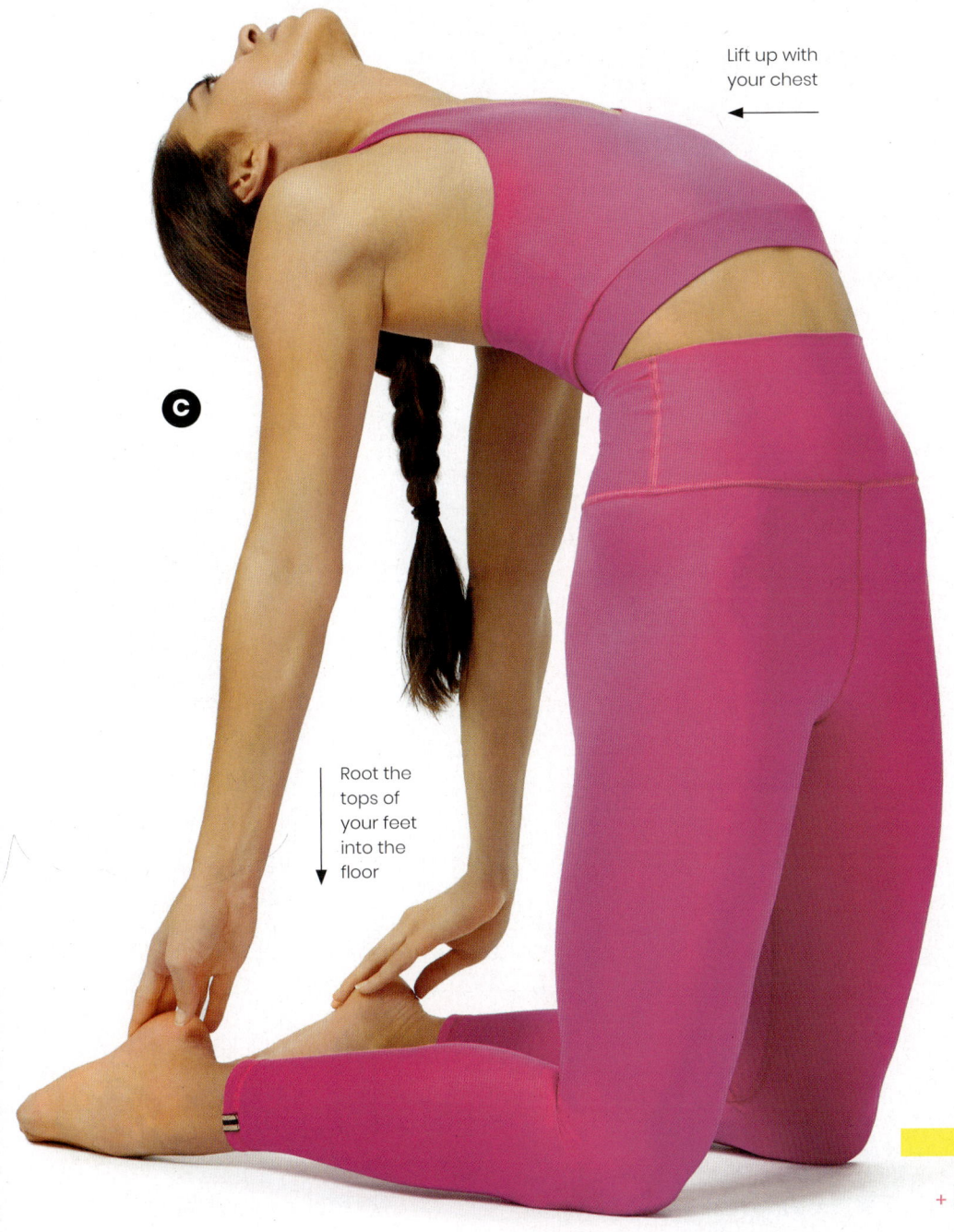

Lift up with your chest

TIP
If you're a beginner, keep your chin tucked in and look forwards.

Root the tops of your feet into the floor

Benefits

+ Strengthens your back
+ Improves your posture
+ Stretches your chest, core and hips
+ Boosts your confidence

CAT POSE
Marjaryasana

MOBILITY

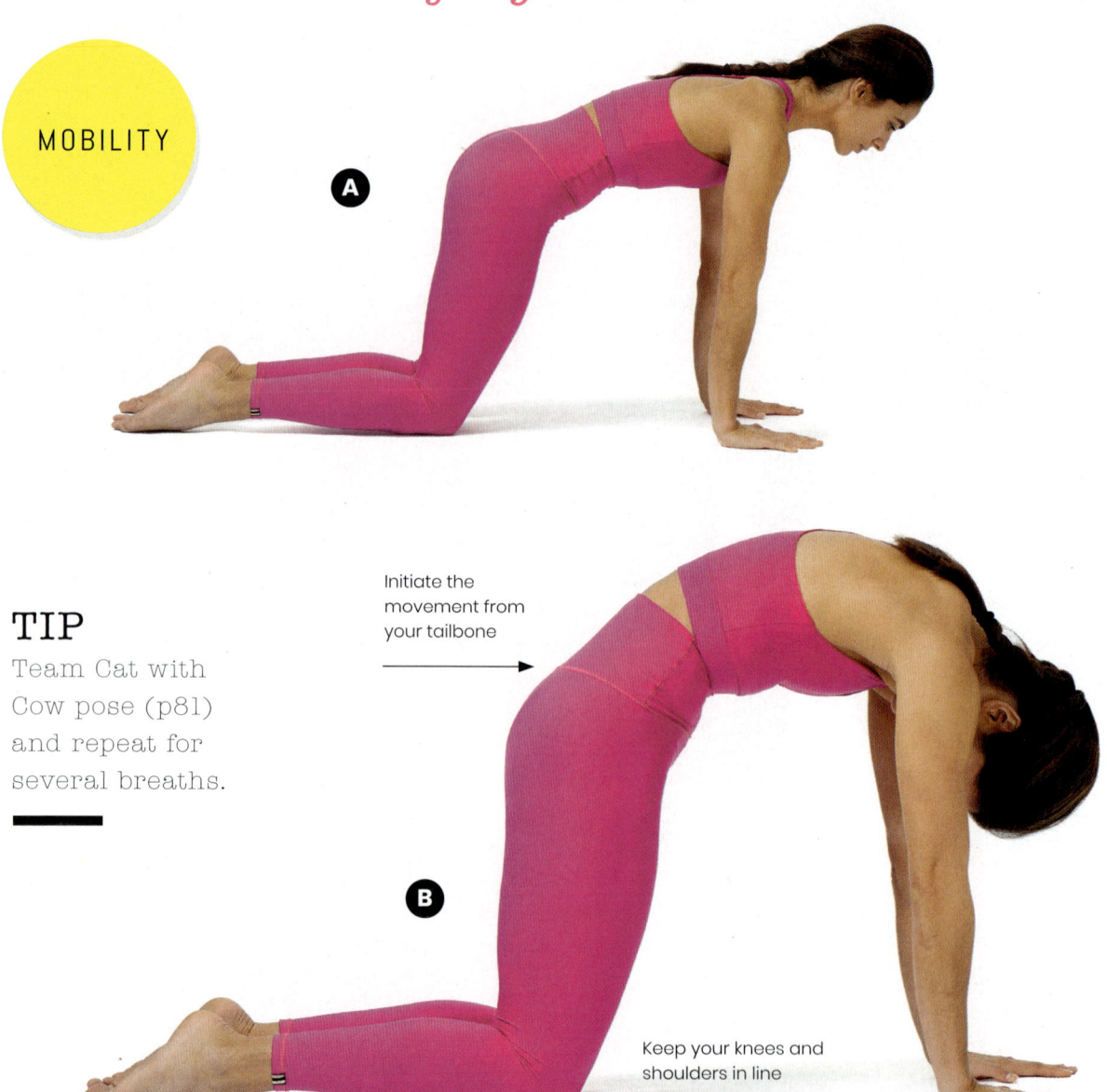

TIP
Team Cat with Cow pose (p81) and repeat for several breaths.

Initiate the movement from your tailbone

Keep your knees and shoulders in line

■ Begin on all-fours with your knees beneath your hips, hands beneath your shoulders and fingers spread (A).
■ Exhale and root through your fingers and the tops of your toes as you release your tailbone and head to the floor and round your spine towards the ceiling (B).
■ Press the floor away with your hands and feel the stretch in your back.
■ Inhale and come back to a neutral position.
■ Repeat several times or inhale into Cow pose (p81).

Benefits

+ Stretches your back
+ Massages your spine
+ Strengthens your hands and wrists
+ Eases stiffness

/ Backbend poses

COW POSE
Bitilasana

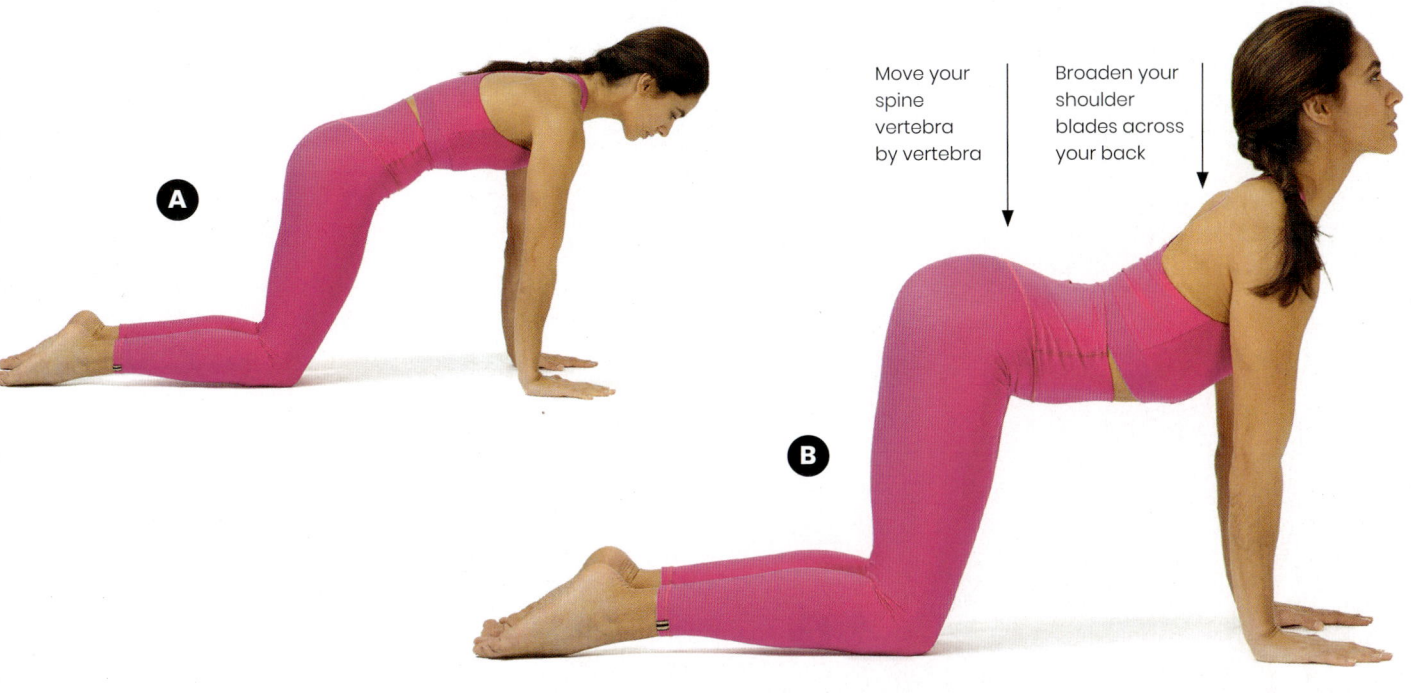

Move your spine vertebra by vertebra

Broaden your shoulder blades across your back

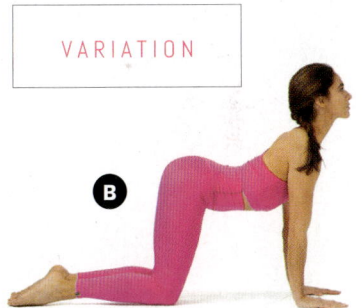

VARIATION

- Begin on all-fours with your knees beneath your hips, hands beneath your shoulders and fingers spread (A).
- Inhale and slowly lift your tailbone and chest up towards the ceiling while releasing your spine and belly down towards the floor into a gentle backbend.
- Draw your shoulders down your back, take your chest forwards and up and gently raise your head to look straight ahead (B).
- Exhale, slowly bringing your spine back to neutral, one vertebra at a time.
- Rest then repeat several times. Or exhale into Cat pose (p80).

Cat/Cow
- For a relaxing stretch or warm-up, combine Cat and Cow into a gentle flow. From Cat pose (A), inhale into Cow (B). Continue alternating between Cat and Cow, instigating the movement from your pelvis and following the natural pattern of your breath. Move vertebra by vertebra in a slow and fluid way. Repeat several times. Try this first thing in the morning, before you go to bed or to counteract sitting at a desk.

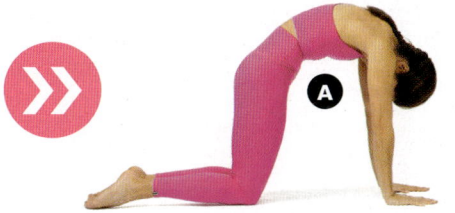

Benefits

+ Stretches your torso and neck
+ Massages your spine
+ Improves mobility

GATE POSE
Parighasana

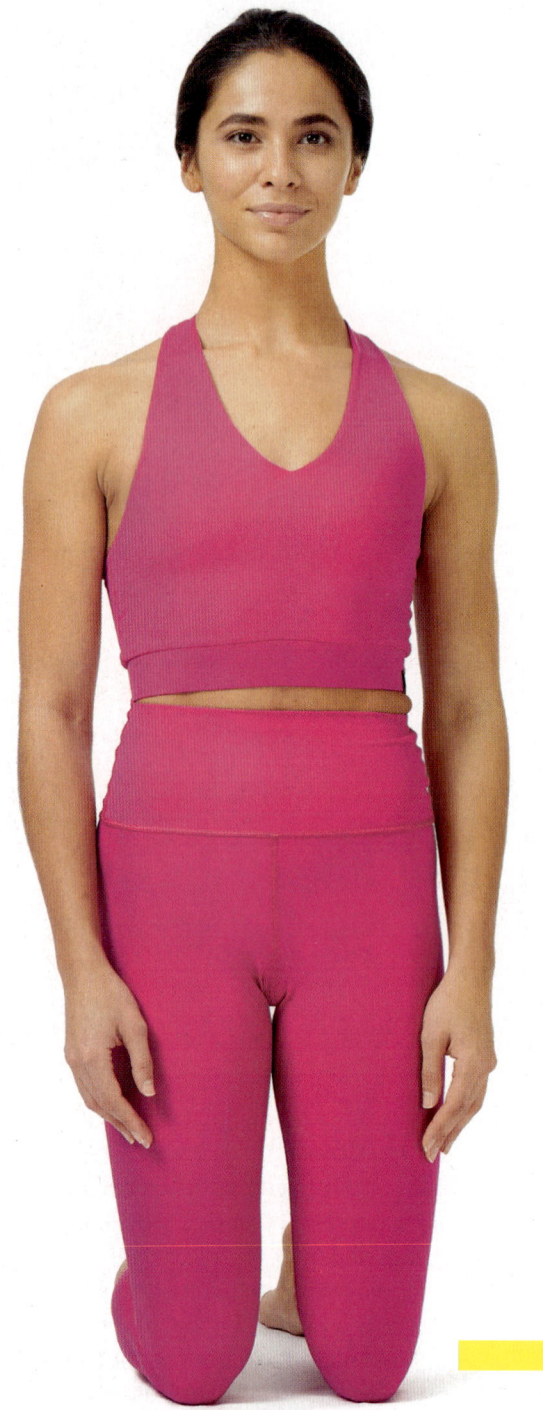

A

Benefits

+ Stretches your spine
+ Opens your chest and side body
+ Stimulates your lungs
+ Improves your balance

STRETCH

■ Start in a kneeling position with your arms relaxed by your sides (A).
■ Once you feel balanced, stretch your right leg out to the side. Gently press your left hip forwards.
■ Take your arms out to the sides, parallel to the floor, palms facing upwards. Inhale and extend the sides of your body, then exhale and lower your arms, placing your right hand on your right leg.
■ Inhale and lift your left arm up and over to the right, alongside your left ear. Gaze up to your arm and extend all the way from your right toes through to your left fingertips (B).
■ Stay in the pose for several deep, slow breaths. On each exhale, feel the stretch deepen in the left side of your body.
■ When you're ready to come out of the pose, inhale and extend through your left arm then exhale and lower it back down.
■ Bring your knees together and repeat on the other side.

Sitting poses

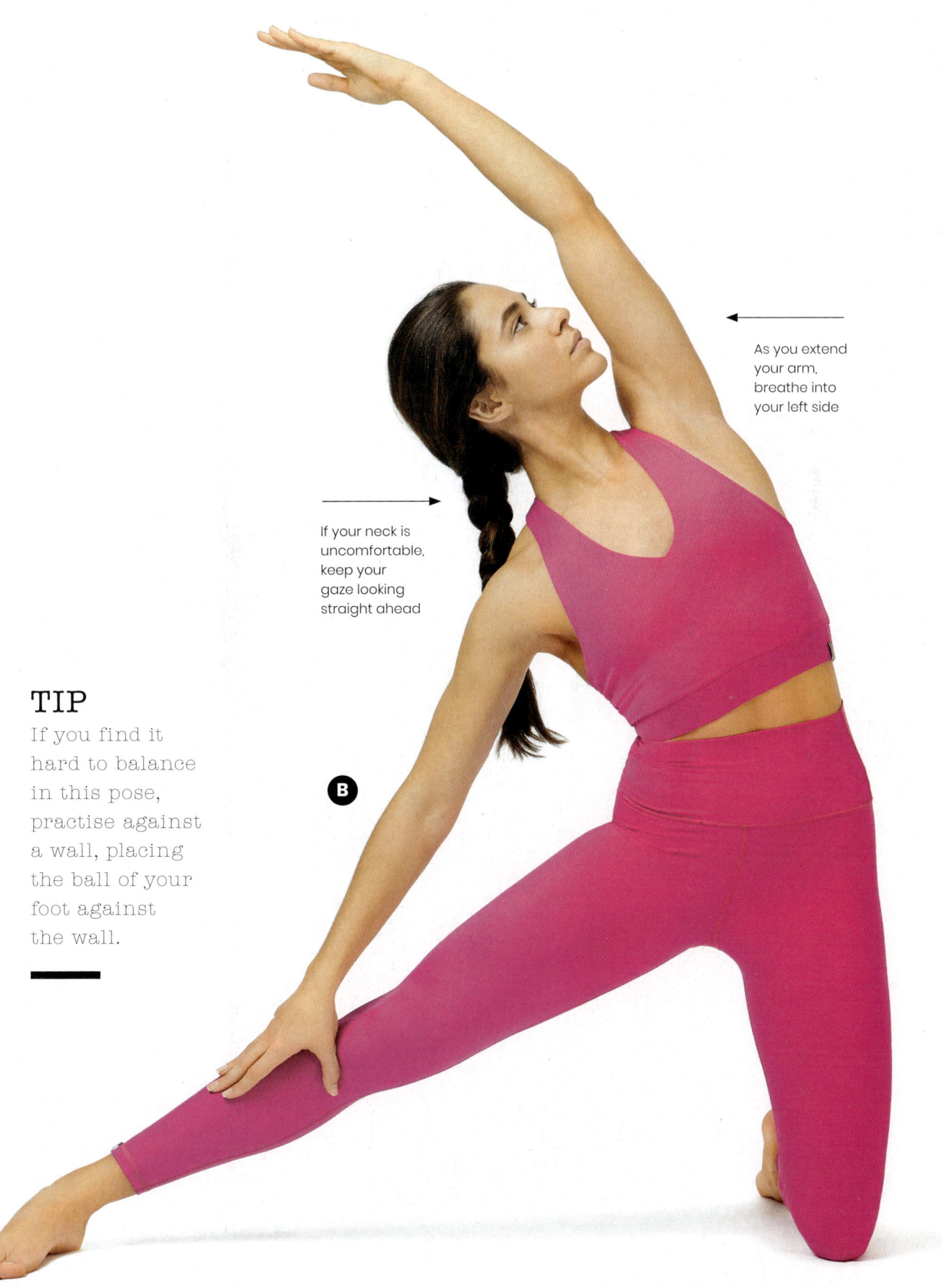

As you extend your arm, breathe into your left side

If your neck is uncomfortable, keep your gaze looking straight ahead

B

TIP
If you find it hard to balance in this pose, practise against a wall, placing the ball of your foot against the wall.

83

COW FACE POSE
Gomukasana

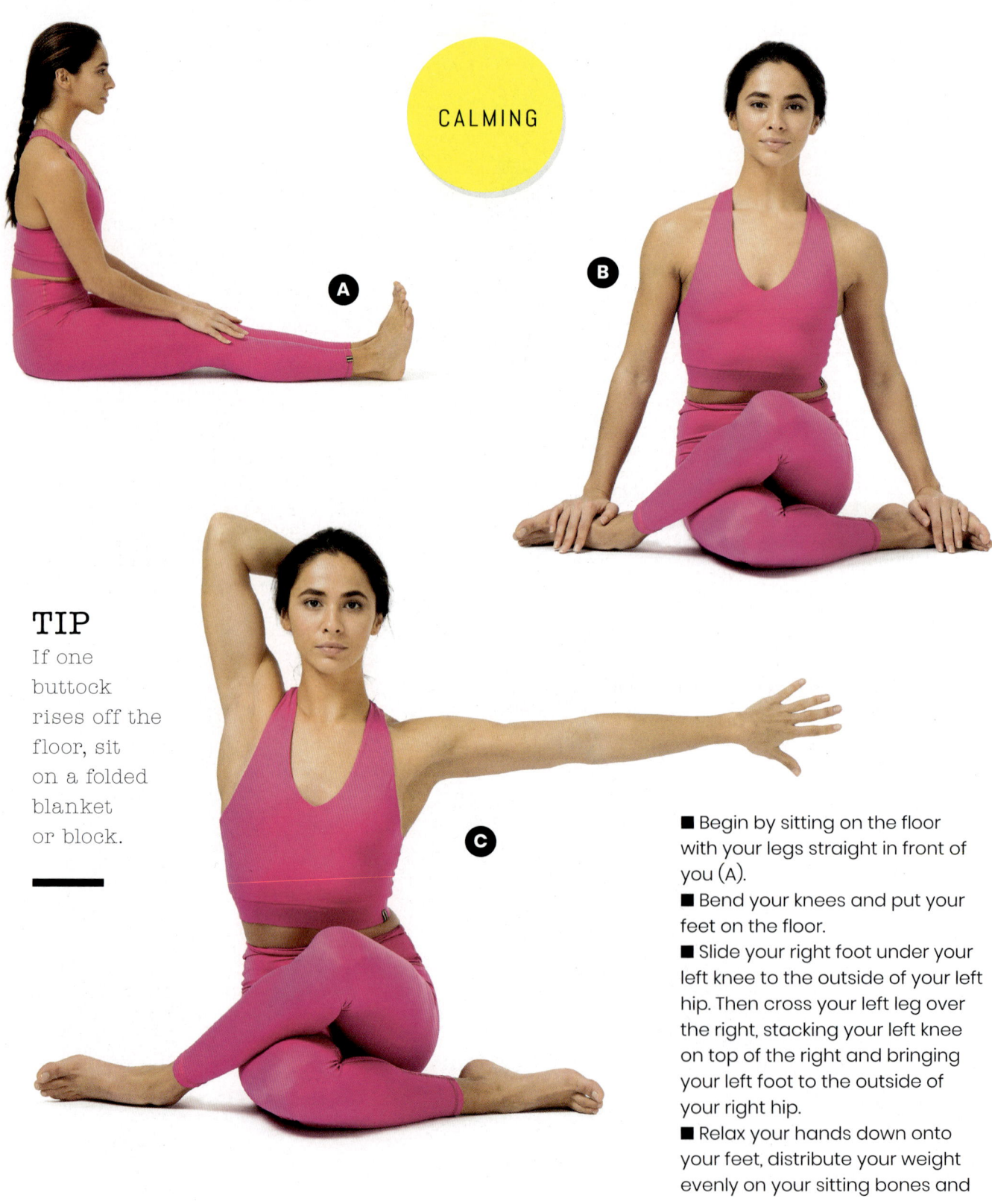

TIP
If one buttock rises off the floor, sit on a folded blanket or block.

■ Begin by sitting on the floor with your legs straight in front of you (A).
■ Bend your knees and put your feet on the floor.
■ Slide your right foot under your left knee to the outside of your left hip. Then cross your left leg over the right, stacking your left knee on top of the right and bringing your left foot to the outside of your right hip.
■ Relax your hands down onto your feet, distribute your weight evenly on your sitting bones and

Sitting poses

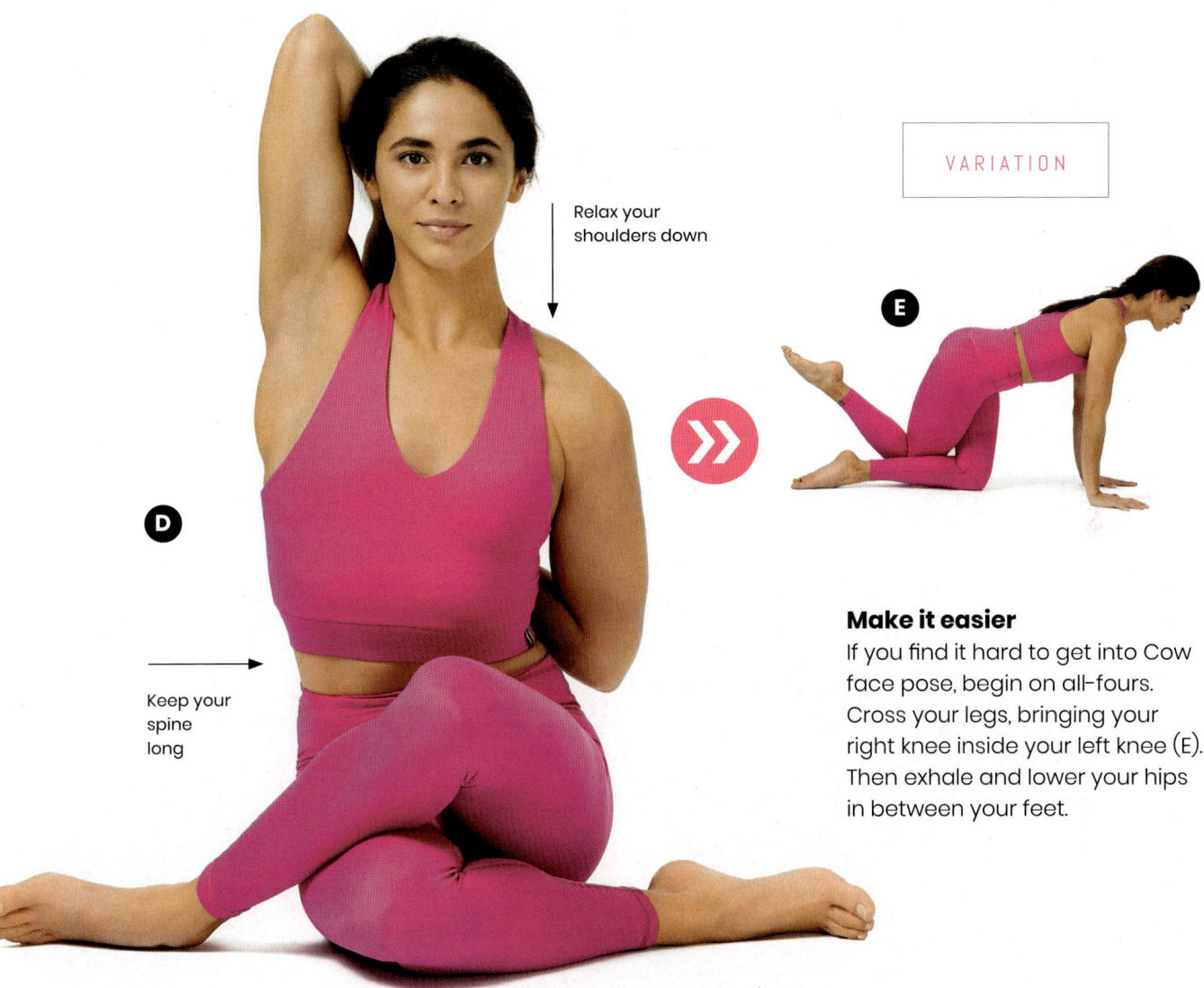

Relax your shoulders down

Keep your spine long

VARIATION

Make it easier
If you find it hard to get into Cow face pose, begin on all-fours. Cross your legs, bringing your right knee inside your left knee (E). Then exhale and lower your hips in between your feet.

let your body relax into the pose (B).
■ Now, inhale and stretch your right arm out to the side. Rotate your palm to face the ceiling, then continue raising your arm until your upper arm is close to your ear.
■ As you exhale, fold your forearm to rest your palm on the centre of your upper back, elbow pointing up.
■ Inhale and raise your left arm out to the side. Turn your palm to face the back of the room (C).

■ Bend your elbow and place the back of your hand between your shoulder blades, taking hold of the fingertips of your left hand (D).
■ Take three to five deep breaths into your belly, rooting through your sitting bones to keep your spine long and your chest open.
■ To come out of the pose, exhale and uncross your legs.
■ Repeat on the other side, switching your arms as well as legs.

Benefits

+ Stretches your hips and ankles
+ Opens your chest
+ Tones your upper arms and shoulders
+ Improves your posture

CHILD'S POSE
Balasana

Lengthen your tailbone away from your pelvis

Broaden your shoulder blades across your back

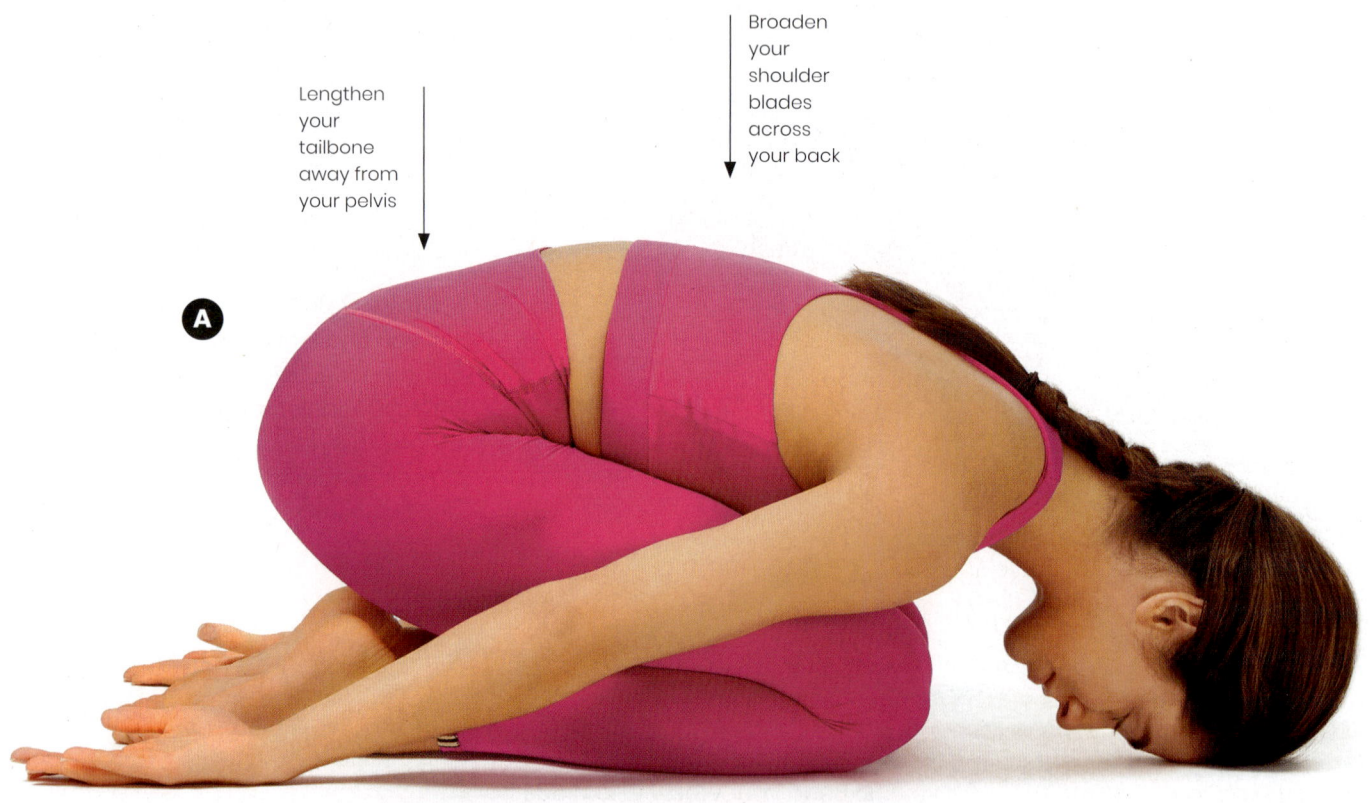

A

TIP
If you struggle to get your forehead to the floor, rest it on a bolster or brick.

Sitting poses

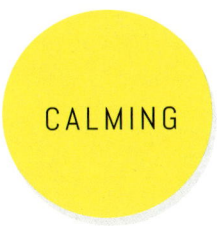

CALMING

- Start in kneeling position. Draw your knees apart and bring your big toes together, heels wide apart. Sit back onto the soles of your feet.
- Resting your palms on your thighs, inhale and root into your sitting bones, lengthening your spine. Exhale and slowly bring your torso down between your thighs.
- Lay your hands on the floor by your sides, palms facing up and let your shoulders release down to the floor.
- Exhale and lower your head to rest your forehead on the floor. Gently close your eyes (A).
- Breathe deeply into the back of your ribs, sinking into the mat on each exhale.
- Stay here for up to a few minutes.
- When you're ready to come out, exhale and use your hands to bring you up to a siting position. Pause for a moment to absorb the benefits.

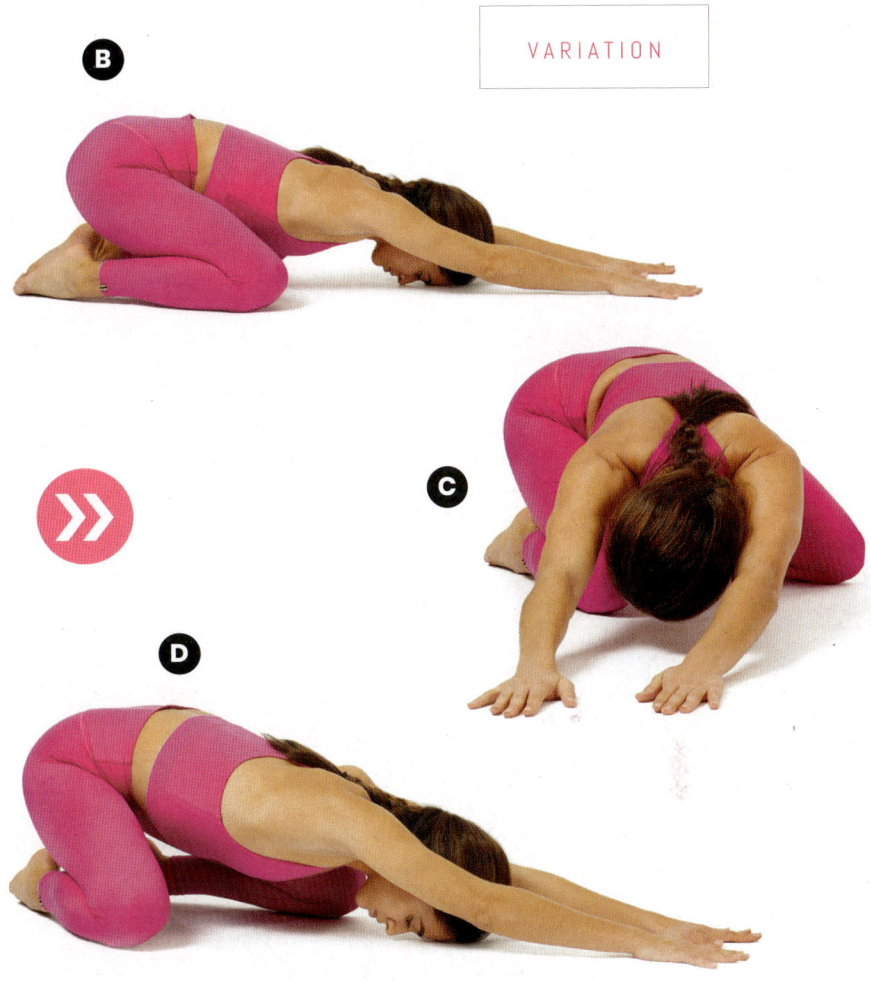

VARIATION

Benefits

+ Relieves stress
+ Calms your mind
+ Rests your body
+ Stretches your hips and thighs

Stretch it out

- For a relaxing stretch, try Extended child's pose. From kneeling, draw your knees apart and bring your big toes together, heels wide apart. Sit back onto the soles of your feet. Exhale and slowly walk your hands forwards, lowering your torso between your thighs. Take your hands shoulder-width apart, palms facing down, fingers spread. Root your hands into the floor, keeping your elbows off the floor and slide your shoulder blades down your back. Exhale and rest your forehead on the floor. Gently close your eyes (B). Next, walk your hands slowly round to the right. Rest here, breathing into the left side of your body (C). Then walk your hands round to the left side and rest here, breathing into the right side of your body (D). Finally, gently walk your hands back to centre and rest for a few breaths.

BANANA POSE
Bananasana

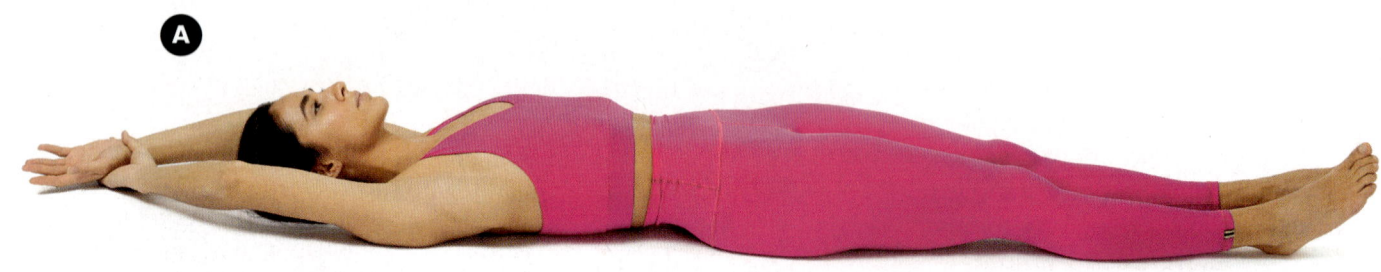

TIP
Try crossing your ankles in the full pose to keep your legs in place.

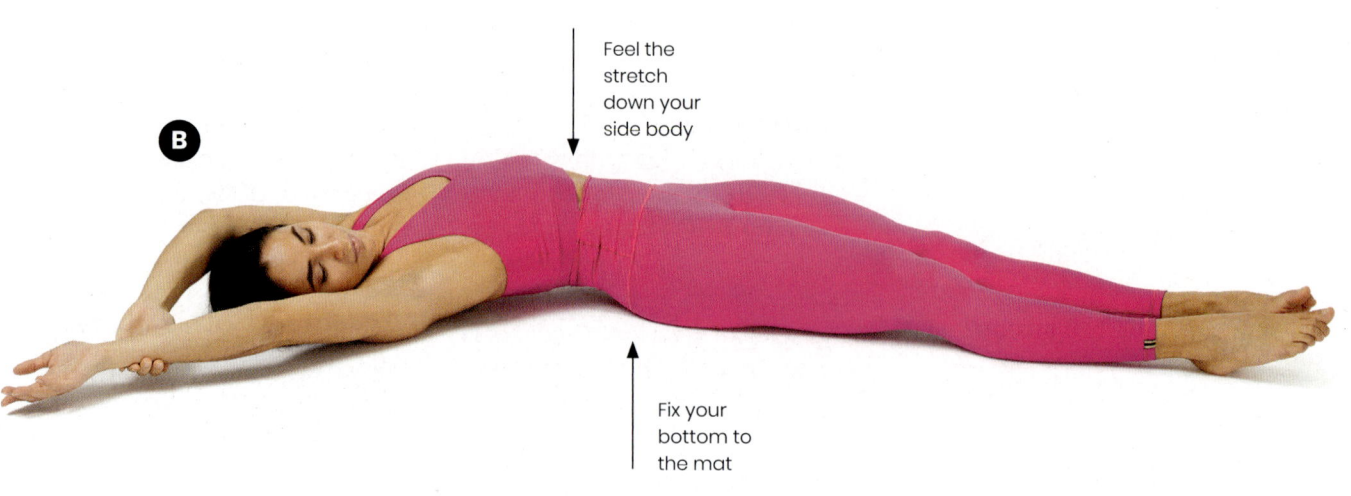

Feel the stretch down your side body

Fix your bottom to the mat

Reclining poses

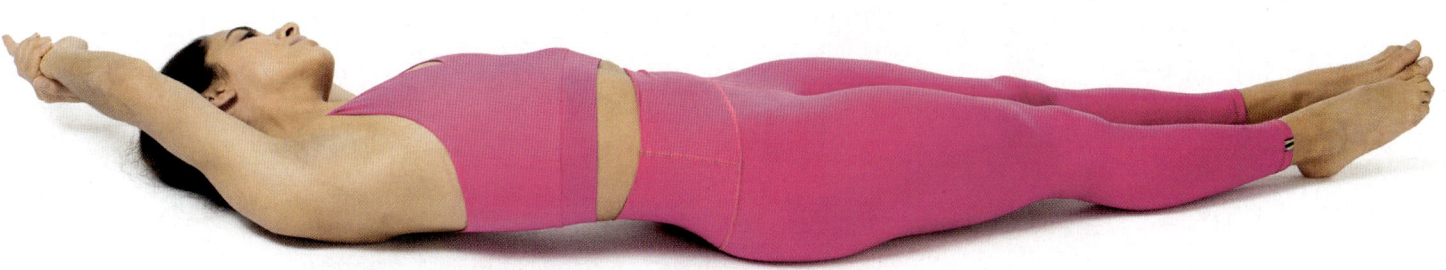

STRETCH

- Lie down on your back with your legs straight and arms relaxed by your sides. Inhale and raise your arms overhead, then clasp your wrists (A).
- Anchor your bottom to the floor and carefully move your legs to the right.
- Next, keeping your bottom anchored to the floor, gently bring your upper body to the right by bending your spine to the side (B).
- Breathe into your left side, feeling the stretch along your left ribs, shoulders, arms, hips and thighs.
- Stay here for up to a minute, breathing gently and deeply. As your body opens, you can move your feet and upper body further to the right.
- When you're ready to come out of the pose, slowly bring your body back to vertical and exhale your arms down to the start position.
- Pause for a few breaths, then repeat on the other side (C).
- When you've completed the pose on both sides, rest in the start position for a few moments to absorb the benefits.

Benefits

+ Works your spine
+ Stretches your side body
+ Stretches your arms and shoulders
+ Tones your core

RECLINING HAND-TO-BIG-TOE POSE
Supta padangusthasana

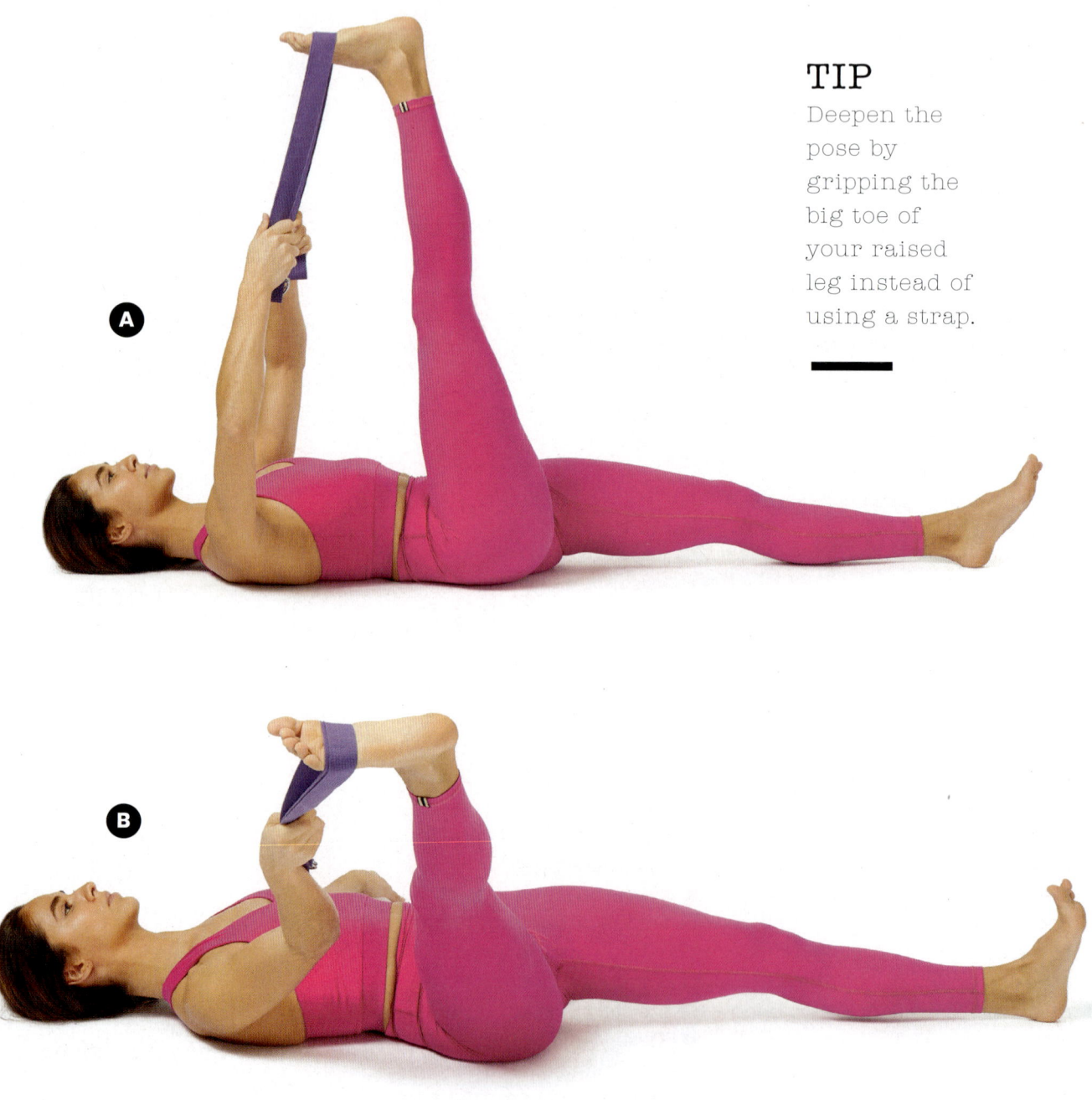

TIP
Deepen the pose by gripping the big toe of your raised leg instead of using a strap.

Reclining poses

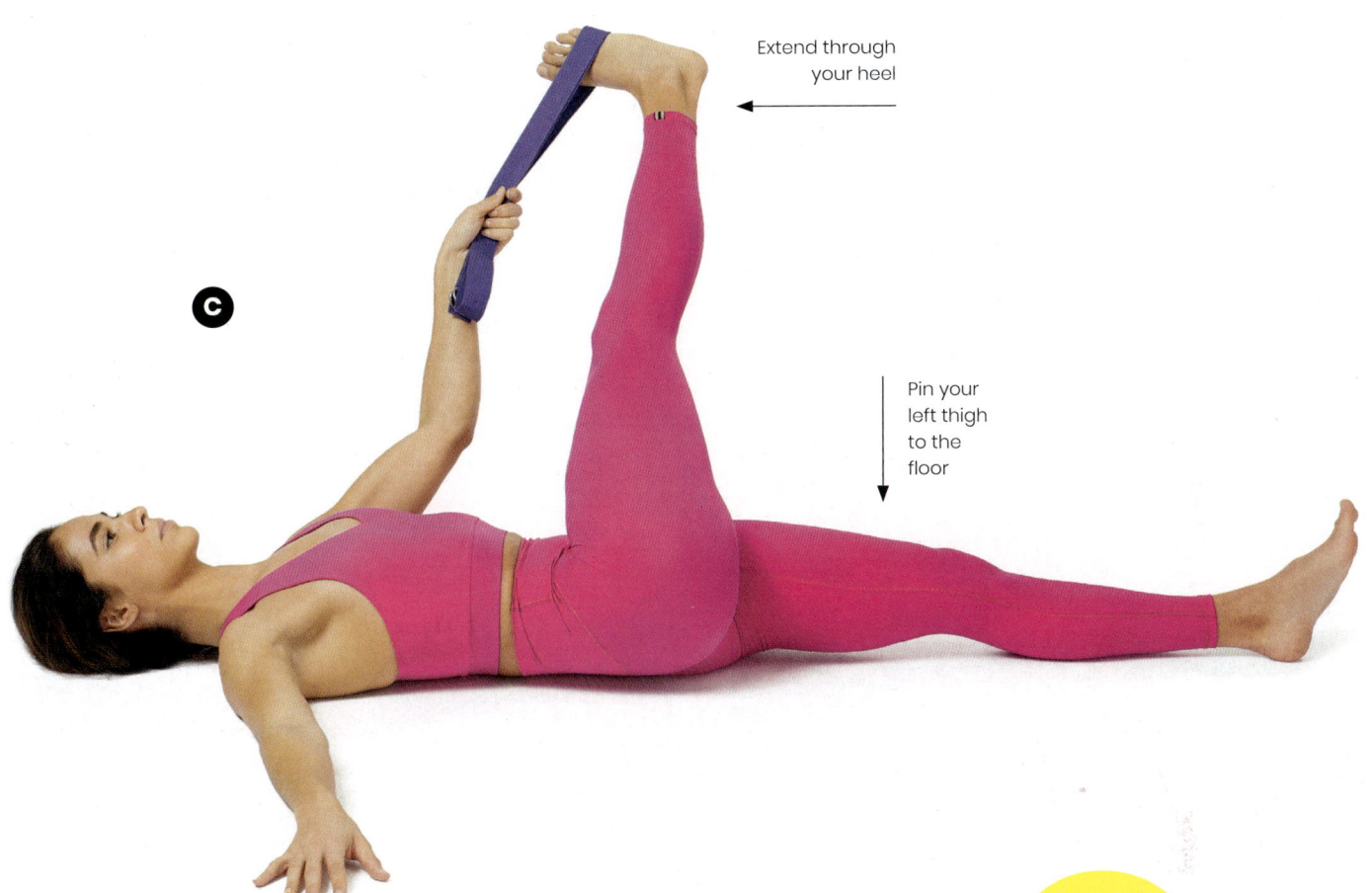

Extend through your heel

Pin your left thigh to the floor

C

- Lie on your back with legs straight and arms relaxed by your sides.
- Bend your right knee and hug it in to your chest with your arms. Take a few, relaxed breaths here.
- Now loop a strap around the arch of your right foot and hold the strap in both hands.
- Inhale and slowly straighten your right leg, pressing your your right heel up towards the ceiling. Walk your hands up the strap until your elbows are straight (A).
- Broaden your shoulders across your back and press your shoulder blades into the floor. On each exhale, draw your foot closer to your head.
- Stay here for five, deep breaths.
- Next, rotate your right leg so that your toes point out to the right side (B).
- Relax your shoulders down away from your ears, keep your lower leg engaged and your left hip down. Take five slow breaths here.
- Once ready, inhale and bring your right leg slowly back to the centre. Take a couple of slow breaths, then release your leg down to the floor.
- Repeat on the other side.
- If it feels comfortable, you can increase the stretch. Hold the strap with your left hand and take your right arm out to the side at shoulder level (C).

STRETCH

Benefits

+ Stretches your hips and hamstrings
+ Relieves backache
+ Strengthens your knees
+ Improves your digestion

CORPSE
Savasana

TIP
Cover yourself with a blanket to stay warm during this pose.

Let your thoughts float away

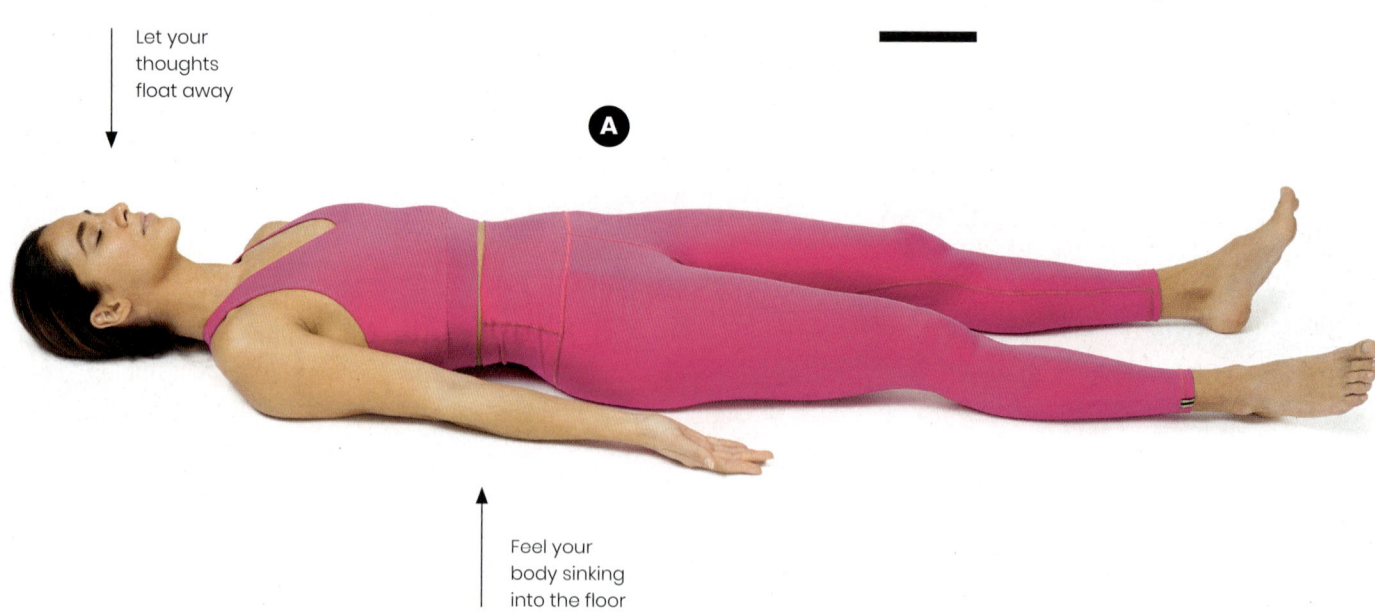

Feel your body sinking into the floor

RELAXING

- Lie on the floor with your legs out in front of you and your feet hip-distance apart.
- Gently release your lower back into the floor. Relax your arms down by your sides with your palms upturned. Gently close your eyes.
- Breathe gently into your belly. On each exhale, let your body sink further into the floor, and feel any tension melt away.
- Relax your neck and shoulders, soften your jaw, let your eyelids go heavy and feel your eyes sink into your head (A).
- Rest in the pose for five to 10 minutes, breathing gently and letting your thoughts drift away.
- When you're ready to come out of the pose, gently start to move your body, wriggling your fingers and toes and slowly turning your head from side to side.
- Roll over to your right side and rest for a moment, then use your hands to come up to a sitting position.

/ Reclining poses

VARIATION

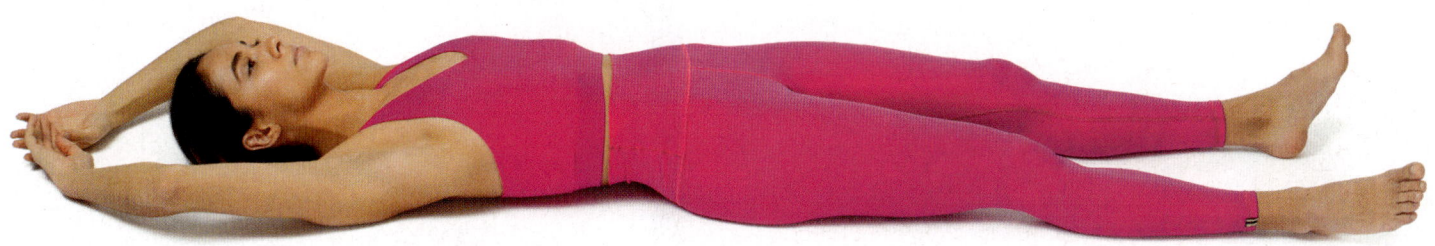

B

Benefits

+ Deeply relaxing
+ Reduces stress and fatigue
+ Lowers blood pressure
+ Aids recovery after practice

Stretch your body

■ To stretch and revive your body, from Corpse pose (A), slowly bring your arms overhead and onto the floor behind you. Stretch your body, extending all the way through from your feet to your fingertips (B).

■ When ready, bring your knees to your chest and rock from side to side to massage your back.

■ Roll over to your right side and rest for a moment, then use your hands to come up to sitting.

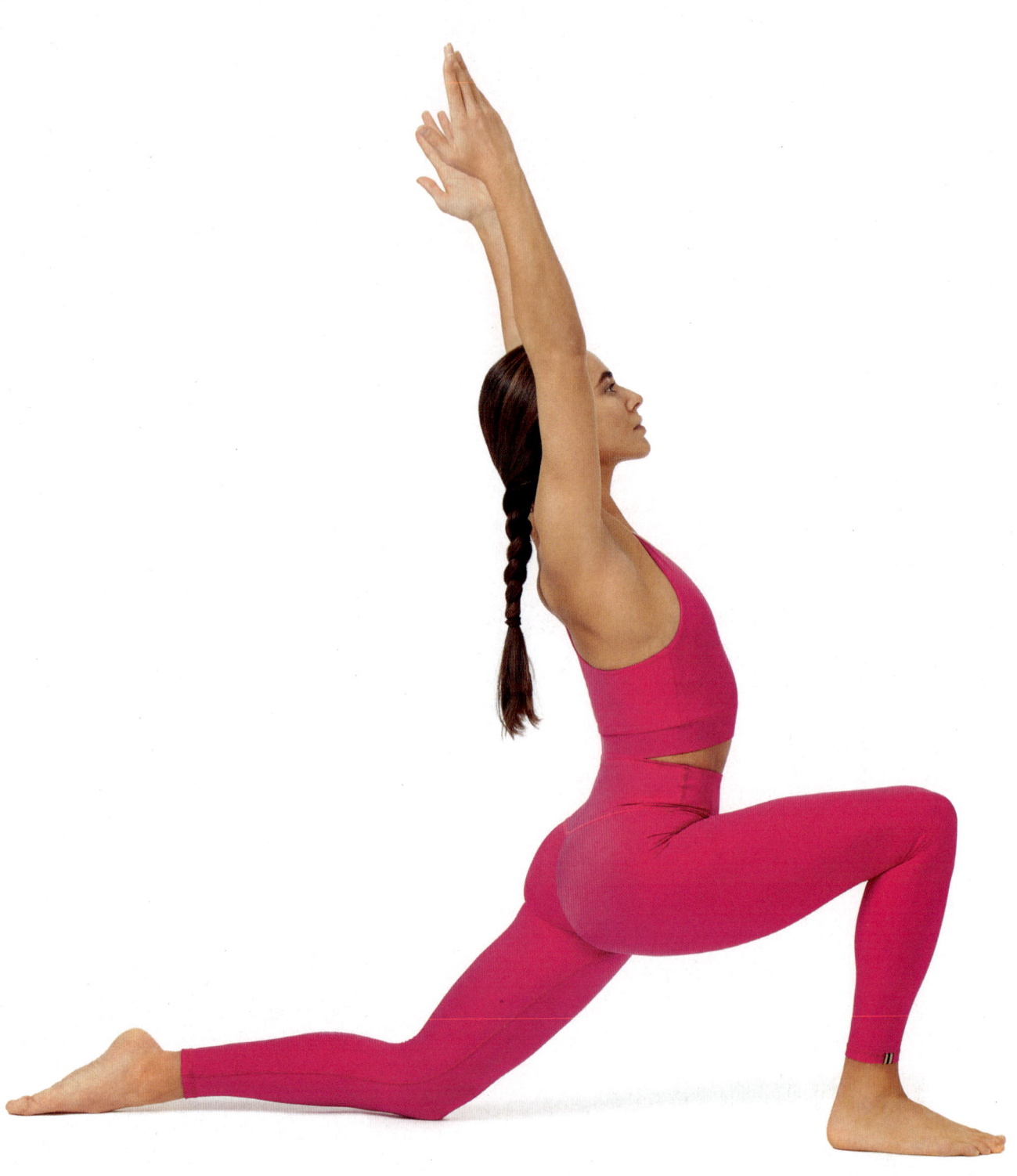

THE SEQUENCES

You've learnt the postures, now it's time to put them together to create your morning sessions. In this section, you'll find a collection of sequences designed by yoga teacher Laura Gate-Eastley to meet your goals, from easing stiff joints and muscles to energising your mind for the day ahead. Begin with some warm-up moves (p96) and Sun salutations (p102) to prime your body, then choose the sequence that's best for you. Go slowly at first to familiarise yourself with the moves, then work more deeply. Let's go!

Wake up YOUR BODY

Ease out morning stiffness and prepare to practise yoga with these simple warm-up moves

Does your body feel stiff and creaky when you get up in the morning? Doing some gentle mobility moves and stretches is the perfect way to wake up your joints and muscles for the day ahead. It's also vital preparation for your morning yoga practice, to ensure you get the most out of your session and avoid injury.

Warming up your muscles and gently opening your joints before you begin your session will help you enjoy doing the poses and sequences more – and make them feel easier too! In the following pages, you'll find a selection of yoga warm-up moves, each targeting different parts of your body. Choose a few moves that will target your areas of concern or prime your body for poses you're planning to practise.

Spending a few minutes warming up also gets you into a more yogic mindset so you can connect to your body and breath during your sessions. You can practise a selection of the moves anytime you're feeling stiff or tired or don't have time for a full yoga session.

Easy twist

Sit in sit in a comfortable cross-legged position and rest the palm of your left hand on the outside of your right knee. Place your right fingertips on the floor behind your hips. Inhale, root through your sitting bones and lift your spine out of your pelvis. Exhale and rotate your spine to the right, from your waist to your upper body. Inhale, lengthen through the crown of your head and exhale further into the twist, turning your head to look over your right shoulder if comfortable for your neck (A). Inhale back to centre and repeat on the other side (B).

Never skip your warm-up – doing yoga with cold muscles can lead to injury!

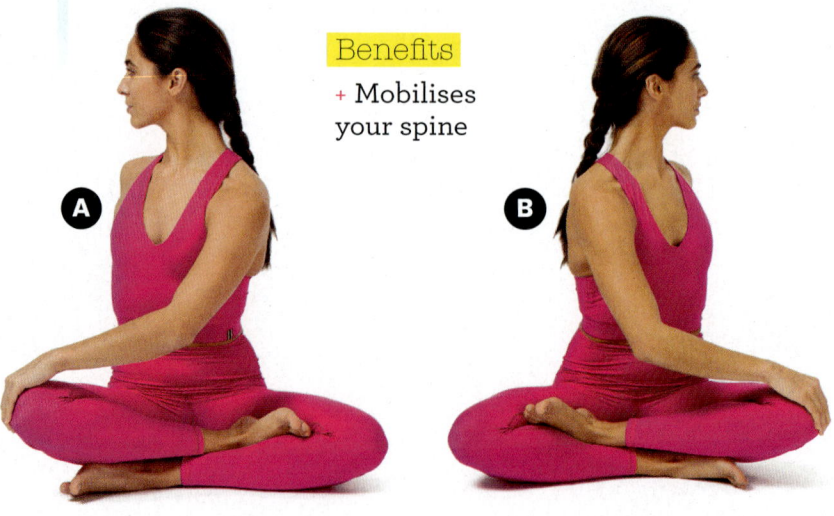

Benefits
+ Mobilises your spine

Warm-up

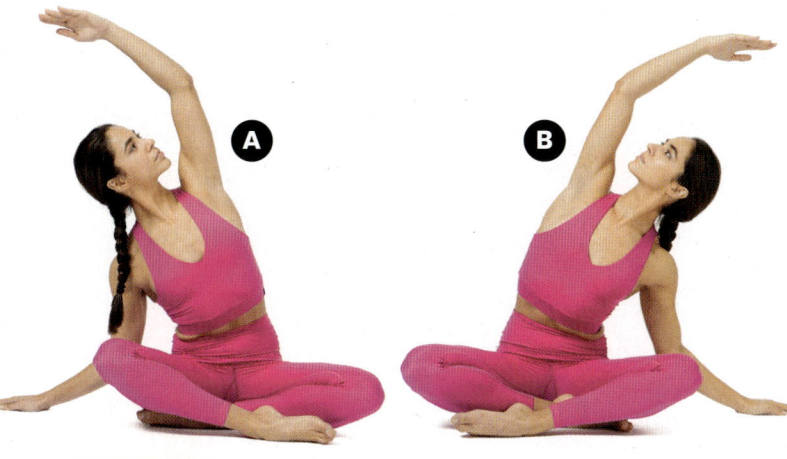

Easy side stretch

Sit in sit in a comfortable cross-legged position and rest your right hand on the floor beside your right hip. Inhale and sweep your left arm overhead. Exhale, then inhale and lift out of your waist to elongate your left side. As you exhale, draw your left hand further over to the right (A). Take one more deep breath here, then inhale back to centre, exhale and lower your arm. Repeat on the other side (B).

Benefits

+ Stretches your side body; deepens your breathing

Head rolls

Sit in sit in a comfortable cross-legged position with your shoulders relaxed. Inhale and bring your left ear as close as possible to your left shoulder (A). Exhale and draw your chin down to your chest (B), then move your right ear as close as possible to your right shoulder (C). Finally bring your head back to an upright position. This is one cycle. Complete five, slow cycles in each direction.

Benefits

+ Releases neck tension; eases stiffness

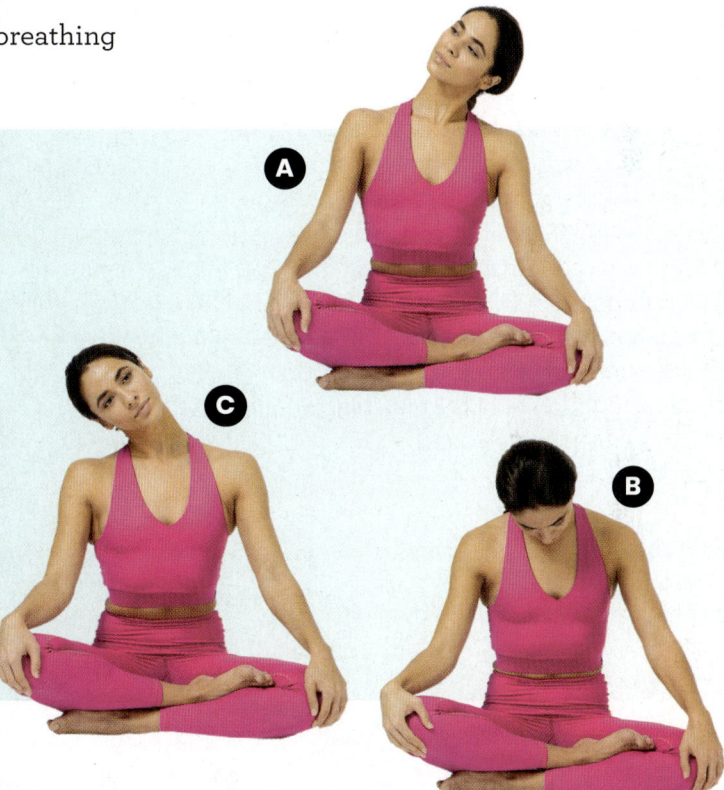

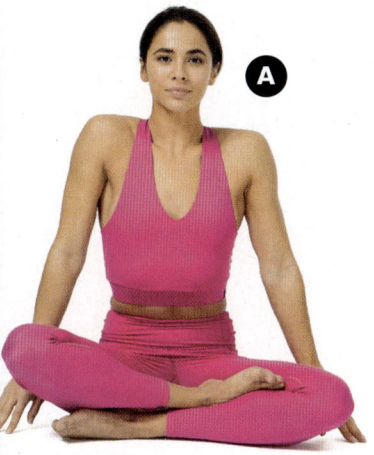
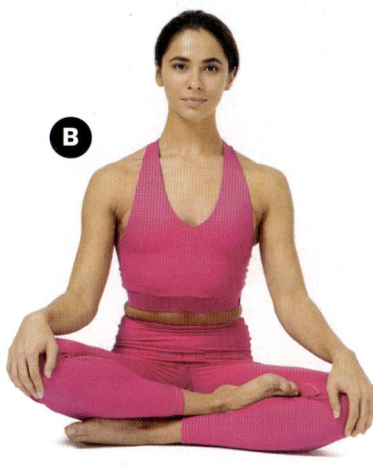

Shoulder shrugs

Sit in sit in a comfortable cross-legged position. Keeping your arms relaxed, inhale and lift your shoulders as close to your ears as you can (A). Exhale and release your shoulders down (B). This is one cycle. Do five cycles, consciously letting go of any tension each time you exhale.

Benefits

+ Releases tension in your shoulders

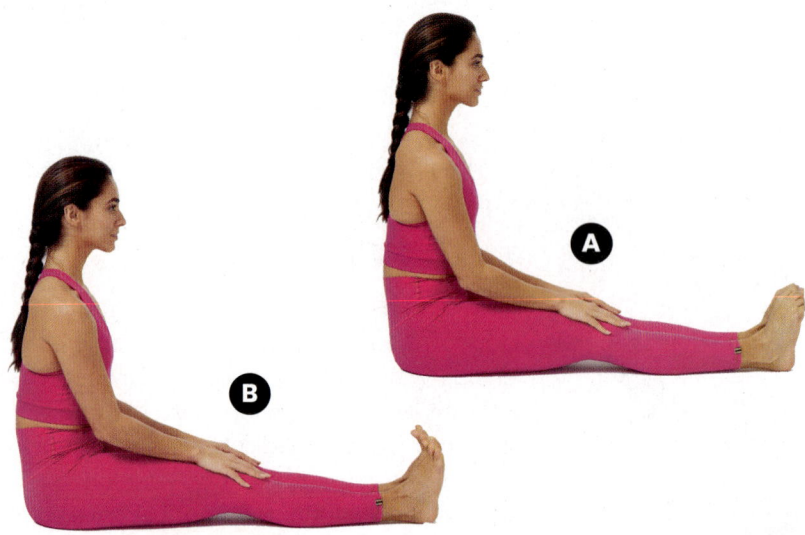

Toe crunches

Sit comfortably with your legs straight out in front of you. Inhale and, as you exhale, bend your toes forwards and squeeze them together, towards the soles of your feet (A). Exhale, release and stretch your toes, separating them as far apart as you can (B). Repeat 10 times.

Benefits

+ Prepares your feet for poses; stretches cramped toes

Elbow circles

Sit in sit in a comfortable cross-legged position and bring your hands to your shoulders (A). Imagine you're drawing large, slow circles out in front of you in a clockwise direction with your elbows, moving them up and forwards (B), down in front of you (C) and then back to the start position. Keep your torso still and your face relaxed. Do five cycles in each direction, keeping your shoulders down and relaxed.

Benefits

+ Stretches your upper arms and shoulders

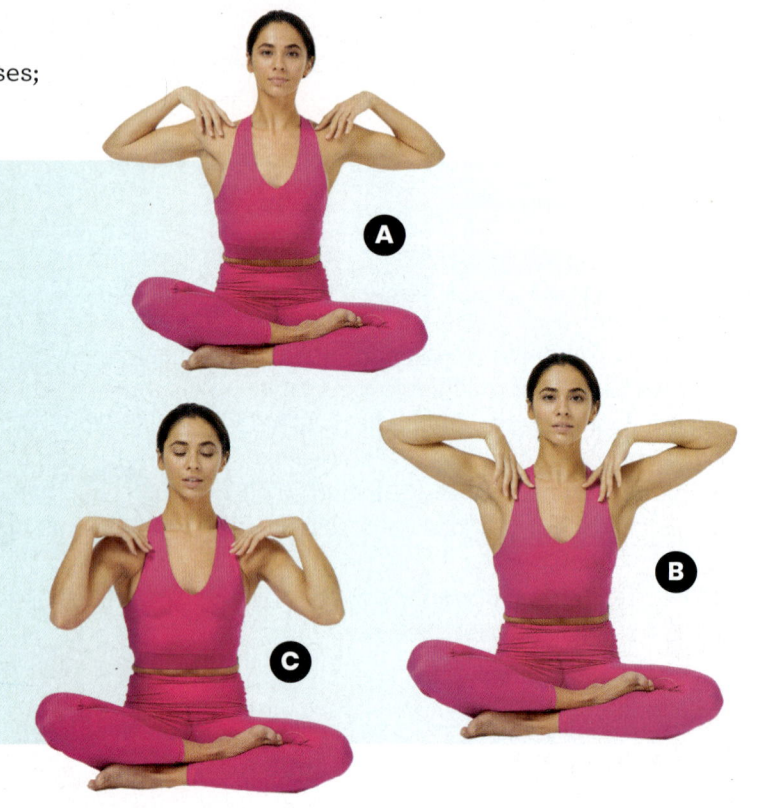

Hand stretches

Sit comfortably with your legs straight out in front of you. Inhale and open your hands as widely as you can, palms forwards and fingers stretched out (A). Exhale and close your fingers to make a tight fist with your thumb inside (B). Repeat 10 times.

Benefits

+ Strengthens your hands; warms up your forearm muscles

Warm-up

Tiger flow

Begin on all-fours in Cat pose (p80) (A). Inhale and lift your right foot back and up towards the ceiling with your knee bent, toes pointing towards your head and spine gently arching (B). Pause, then exhale and bring your knee towards your chest as you arch your spine upwards (C). Move in time with your breath and repeat the move several times.

Benefits
+ Stretches your shoulders and front of your thighs; strengthens your arms

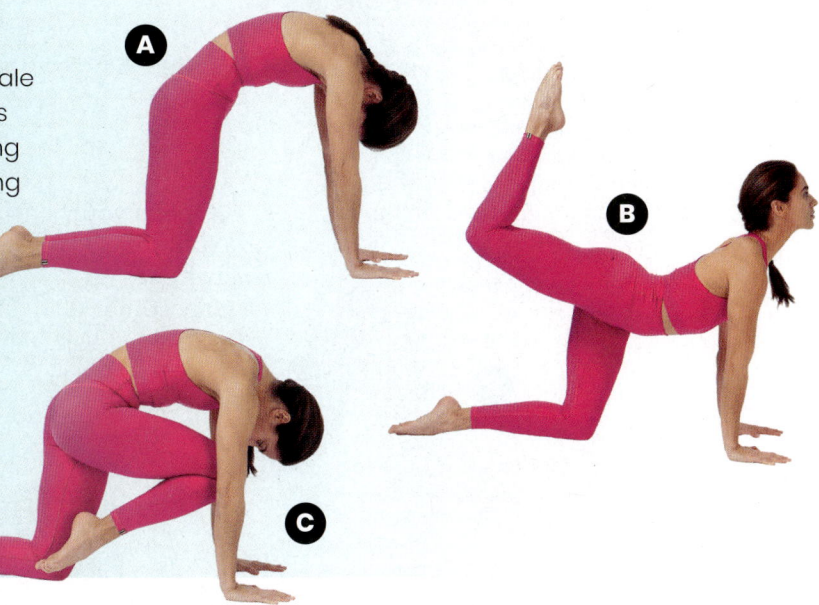

Thread the needle

Begin on all-fours with your shoulders over your wrists and hips over your knees. Inhale, raise your right arm out to the side and overhead (A). Exhale and slide your arm (palm facing up) beneath your torso, extending your right hand under your left arm and out to the side. Take your left hand forwards a few inches, then press it into the floor, bend your left elbow and rest your right shoulder on the floor to deepen the twist (B). Exhale to release, then repeat on the other side.

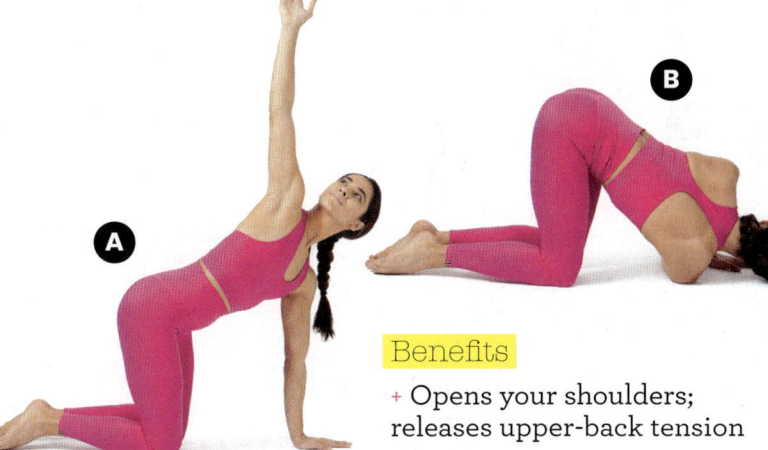

Benefits
+ Opens your shoulders; releases upper-back tension

Bridge

Lie on your back with your knees bent, feet hip-distance apart and parallel, close to your bottom. Rest your arms by your sides, palms facing down (A). Inhale and ground through your feet. Exhale, tilt your tailbone up and slowly lift your bottom and spine up off the floor, vertebra by vertebra, until your weight is on your shoulders. Root through your feet to lift your chest (B). Then reach your hands under your body, clasp your fingers together and draw your shoulders together, lifting your chin slightly away from your chest and pressing your knees away from your chest (C). Take five deep breaths into your belly. Exhale and slowly roll down your spine to rest on the floor.

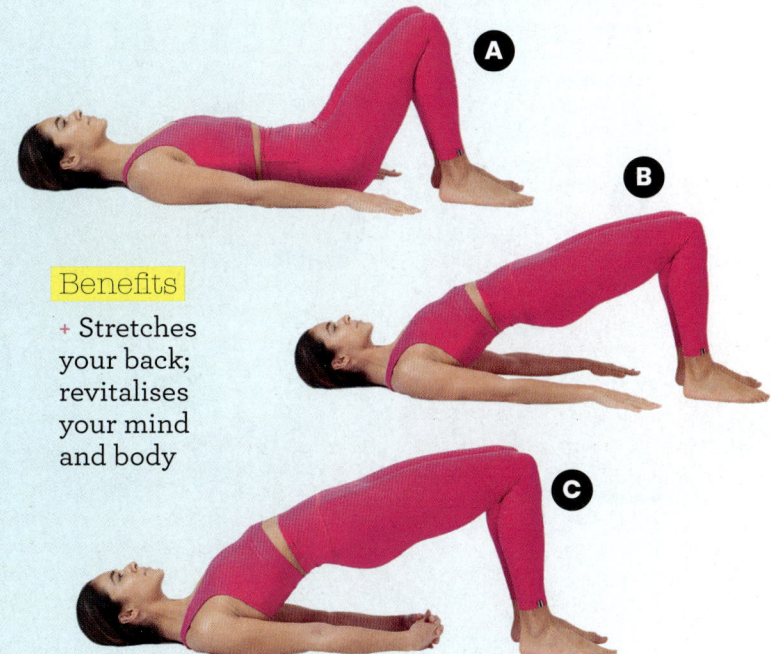

Benefits
+ Stretches your back; revitalises your mind and body

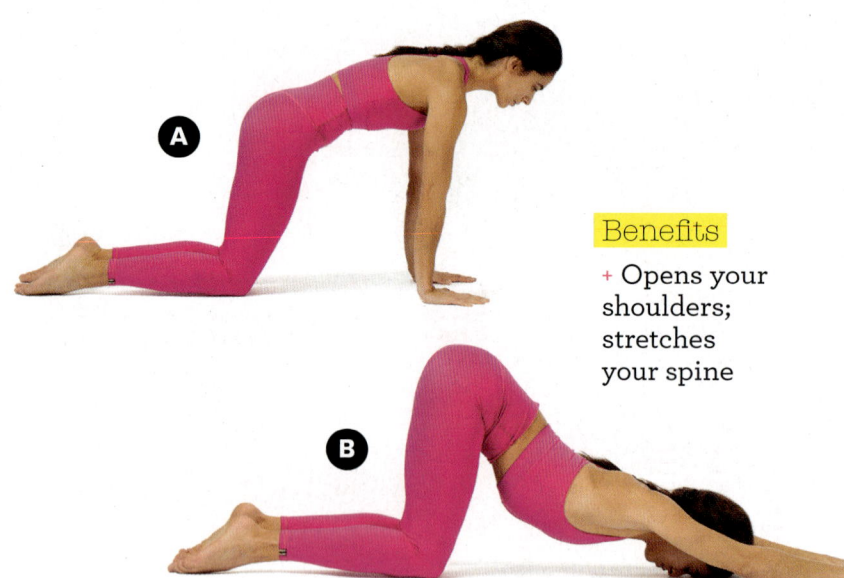

Puppy dog

From all-fours (A), walk your hands forwards a hand's-length or two. Inhale, then exhale and root through your hands as you take your hips back slightly to lengthen your spine. Keeping your arms active and fingers spread, lower your head to the floor (B). Relax your neck and take five deep breaths into your back body. To come out, exhale and walk your hands back in, then come back up to kneeling.

Benefits
+ Opens your shoulders; stretches your spine

Lion's breath pose

Begin on all-fours, your hands under your shoulders and knees under your hips (A). Inhale deeply, then open your eyes and mouth wide, stretch your tongue out, contract the muscles of your throat and exhale slowly, making the sound 'ha' (B). Repeat two or three times, feeling all tension release as you make the roaring noise.

Benefits
+ Wakes up your face; releases tension in your chest

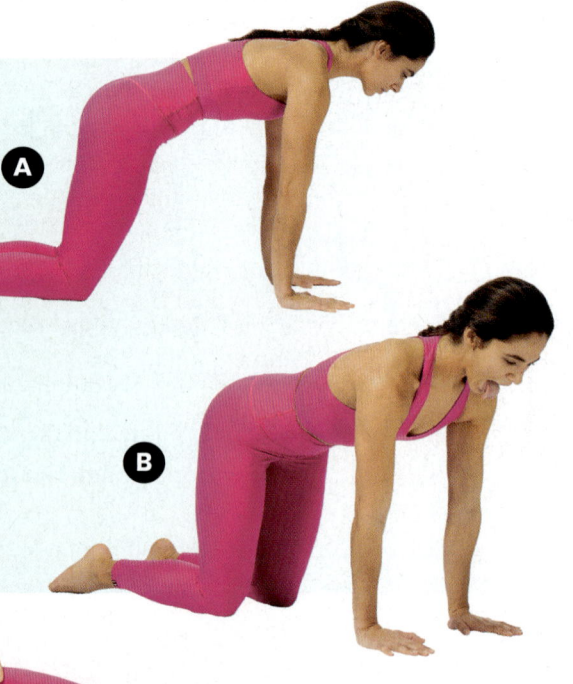

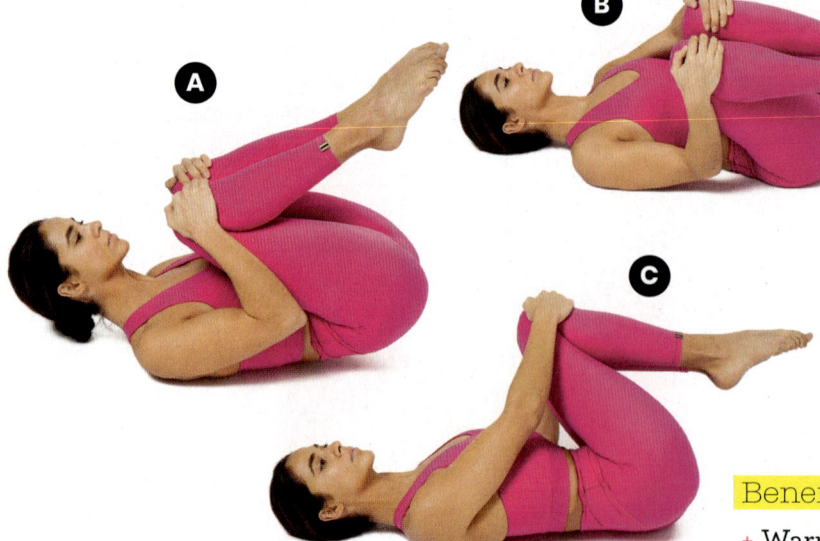

Side rolls

Lie on your back and bring your knees into your chest. Place your hands on your knees and take a few relaxing breaths (A).
Now start to slowly roll your body to the right (B) and left (C) using your breath and core to control the movement. Repeat several times in each direction.

Benefits
+ Warms up your hip joints; releases your body

Warm-up

Eye of the needle

Lie on your back and rest your left ankle on your right thigh. Thread your left hand between your thighs and interlace your fingers behind your right knee (A). If your hands don't reach, wrap a strap around your right thigh. Use your arms to draw your right knee towards your chest as you press your left forearm into your left thigh to open your left hip (B). Take five deep breaths here, then repeat on the other side.

Benefits

+ Opens your hips; releases tight glutes

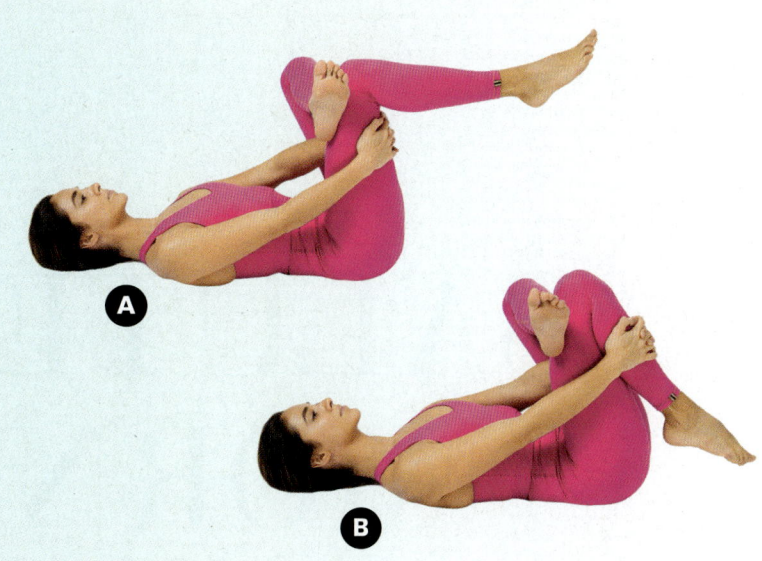

Benefits

+ Releases tension; stretches your inner thighs and back

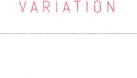

VARIATION

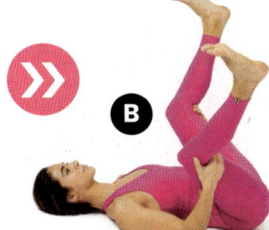

Happy baby

Lie on your back, bend your knees into your belly, then inhale and hold the outsides of your feet. Open your knees, flex your ankles and bring your calves to vertical. Push your feet up into your hands and pull down, feeling the stretch in your inner and outer thighs and the release in your lower back (A). Keeping your chin tucked in and your neck long, draw your shoulders down your back to lengthen your spine. If you can't hold your feet, hold the back of your knees or shins instead (B). Take 10 deep breaths, then rock from side to side to massage your back. Exhale and release back down to the floor.

Spine roll

Lie flat on your back and bend your knees into your chest, holding your knees with your hands (A). Take a breath and then, on an exhale, move your hands to the back of your knees and start to roll backwards (B) and forwards (C) in a rocking motion, keeping your chin into your chest and your core engaged. Repeat up to 10 times, feeling the motion massaging your spine.

Benefits

+ Massages your spine and hips; wakes up your body

SALUTE THE MORNING

Kickstart your day with classic Sun salutation sequences, suitable for every level from beginner to advanced

The perfect way to start your day, Sun salutations are a flowing set of poses co-ordinated with your breath to create a dynamic, energising sequence. One of the foundations of Hatha yoga practice, Sun salutations are often practised in classes as a warm-up for more challenging practice. Performed first thing in the morning, Sun salutations help ease any stiffness and generally wake up your body and mind. Practise them slowly for a deep, mindful stretch; or pick up the pace for a cardio workout that will kickstart your metabolism, burn calories and strengthen your body from top to toe.

HALF SUN SALUTATION

This simple, flowing sequence is ideal for beginners or when you want a gentle start to the day.

How to do it
Begin by grounding yourself in Mountain pose. Then begin the sequence, taking it slowly and following the breathing instructions. Try performing three rounds, then end by resting for a few moments in Mountain to absorb the benefits.

1. **Mountain pose** (p40)
Inhale into...
2. **Extended mountain pose** (p41)
Exhale into...
3. **Standing forward bend** (p42)
Inhale into...
4. **Half-standing forward bend** (p43)
Exhale into...
5. **Standing forward bend** (p42)
Inhale into...
6. **Extended mountain pose** (p41)
Exhale into...
7. **Mountain pose** (p40)

AS YOU PROGRESS, YOU CAN MOVE ONTO SUN SALUTATION A AND B.

Sun saluations

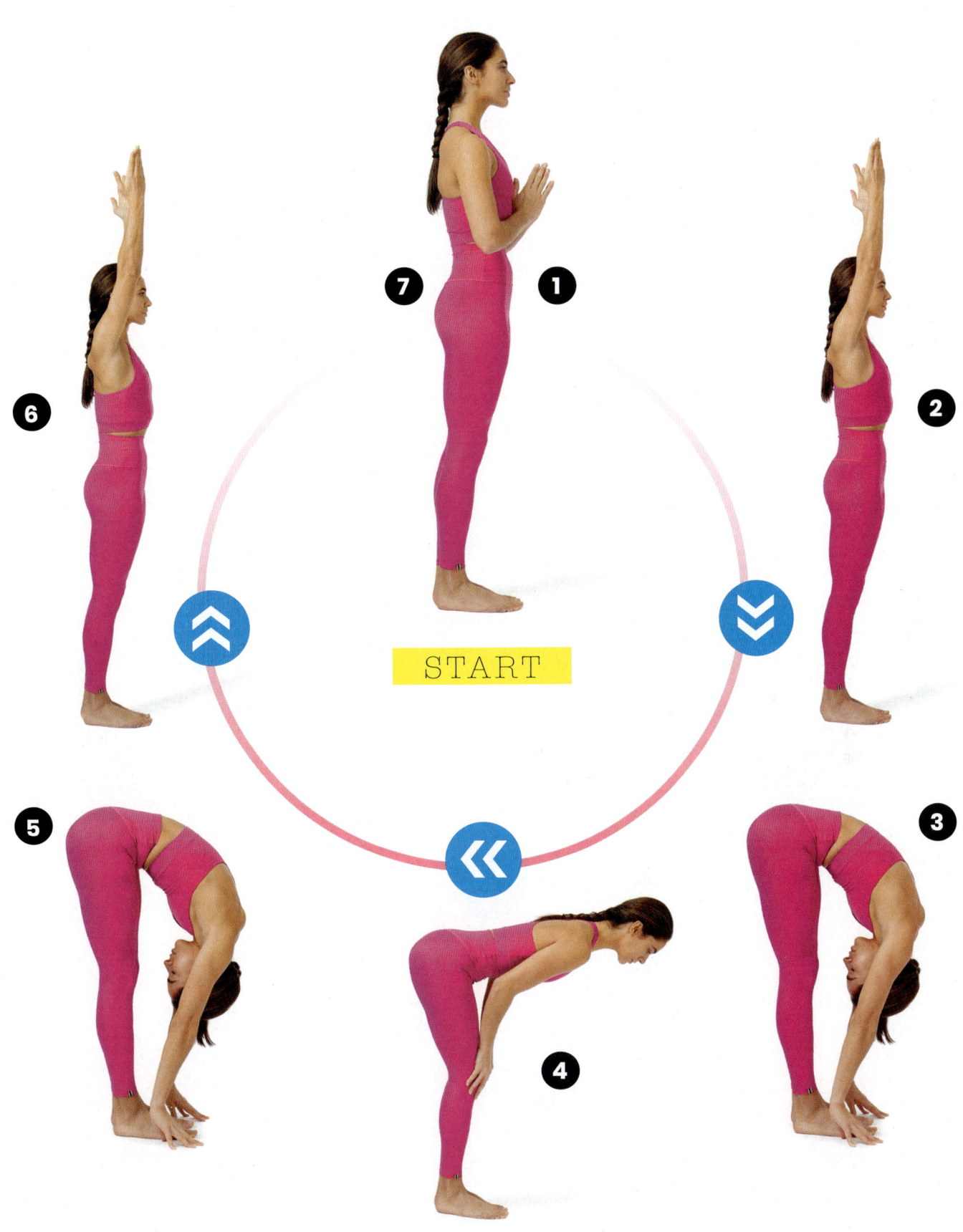

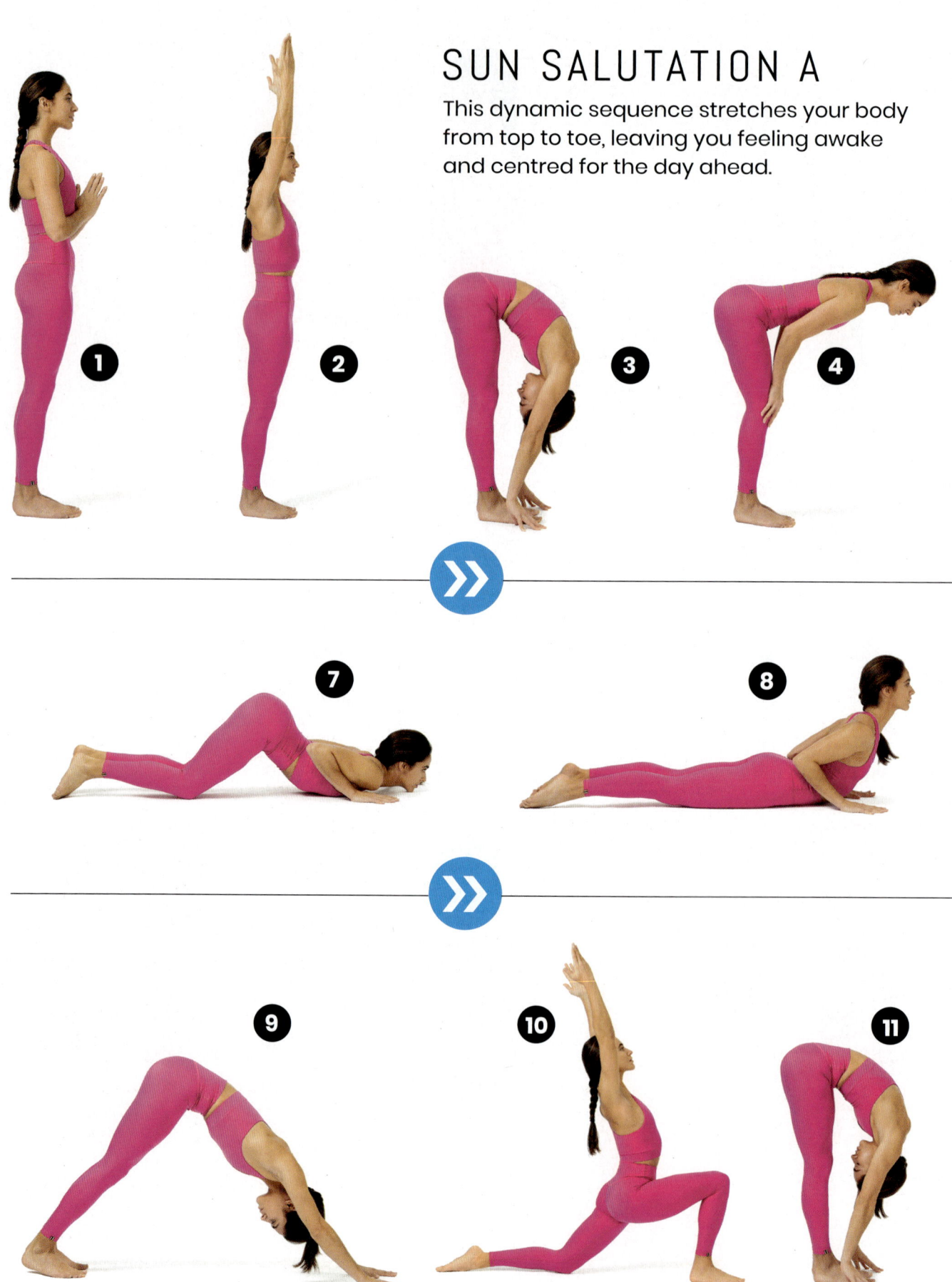

SUN SALUTATION A

This dynamic sequence stretches your body from top to toe, leaving you feeling awake and centred for the day ahead.

Sun salutations

TIP
Beginners, try taking three breaths in each pose.

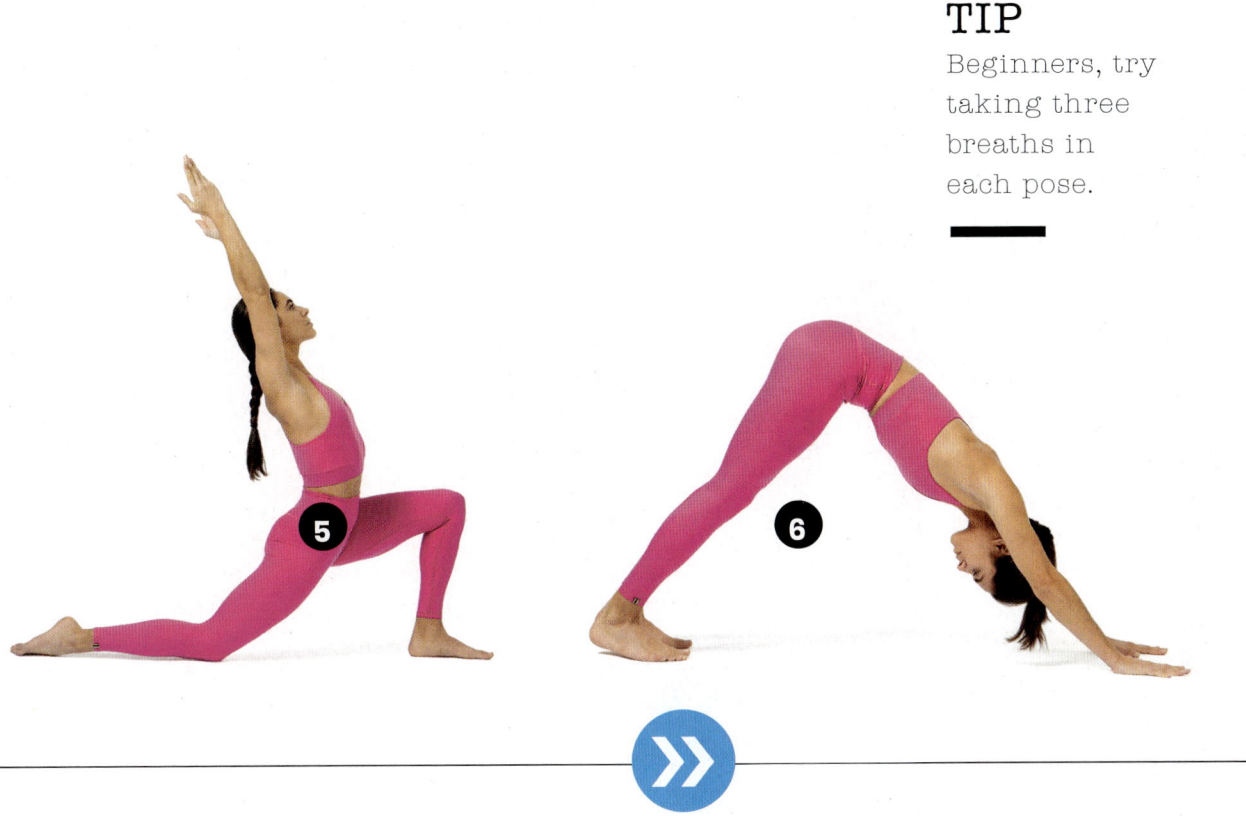

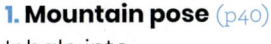

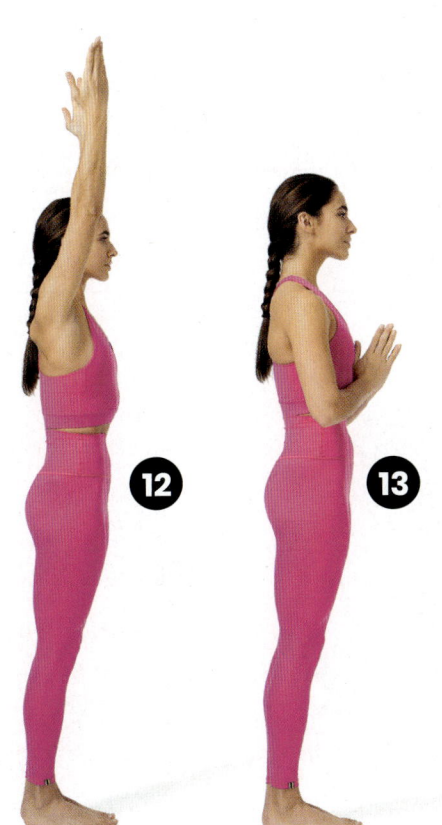

How to do it
Begin by working through the poses slowly in synch with your breath, to create a moving meditation. Once you've got the hang of it, you can pick up the pace to suit your mood.

1. Mountain pose (p40)
Inhale into...
2. Extended mountain pose (p41)
Exhale into...
3. Standing forward bend (p42)
Inhale into...
4. Half-standing forward bend (p43)
Inhale and step your right leg back into...
5. Low lunge (p48)
Exhale and step your left leg back into...
6. Downward-facing dog (p62)
Take five deep breaths, then exhale into...
7. Caterpillar (p73)
Hold your breath as you lower your chest and knees to the floor, then your abdomen, and then inhale into...
8. Cobra (p72)
Exhale and lift back into...
9. Downward-facing dog (p62)
Inhale as you step your right foot forwards into...
10. Low lunge (p48)
Exhale and step your left foot forwards into...
11. Standing forward bend (p42)
Inhale, taking your arms out to the side and overhead to...
12. Extended mountain pose (p41)
Exhale your arms out to the side and into...
13. Mountain pose (p40)

Repeat the sequence, leading with your left leg. This completes one round.

105

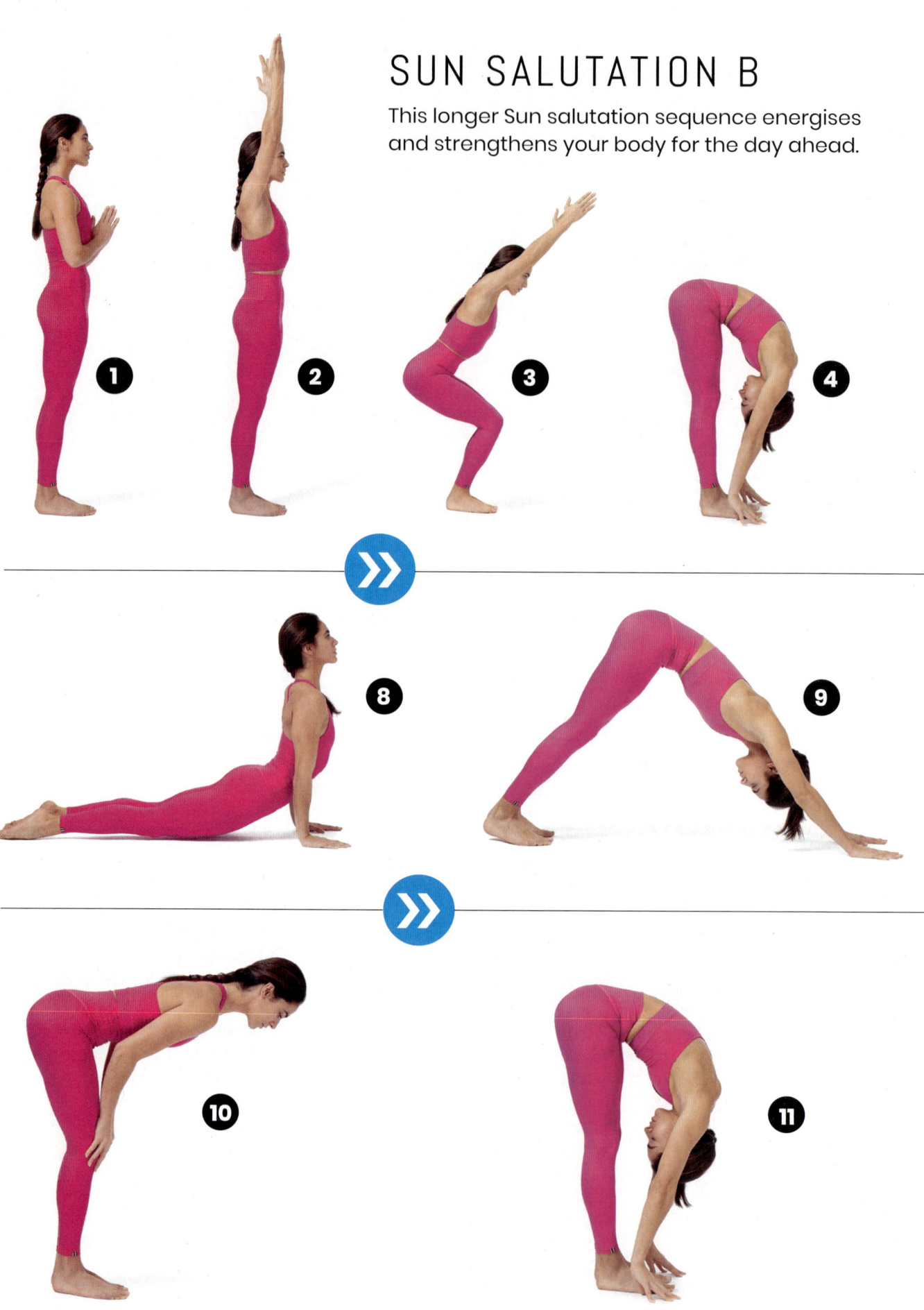

SUN SALUTATION B

This longer Sun salutation sequence energises and strengthens your body for the day ahead.

Sun saluations

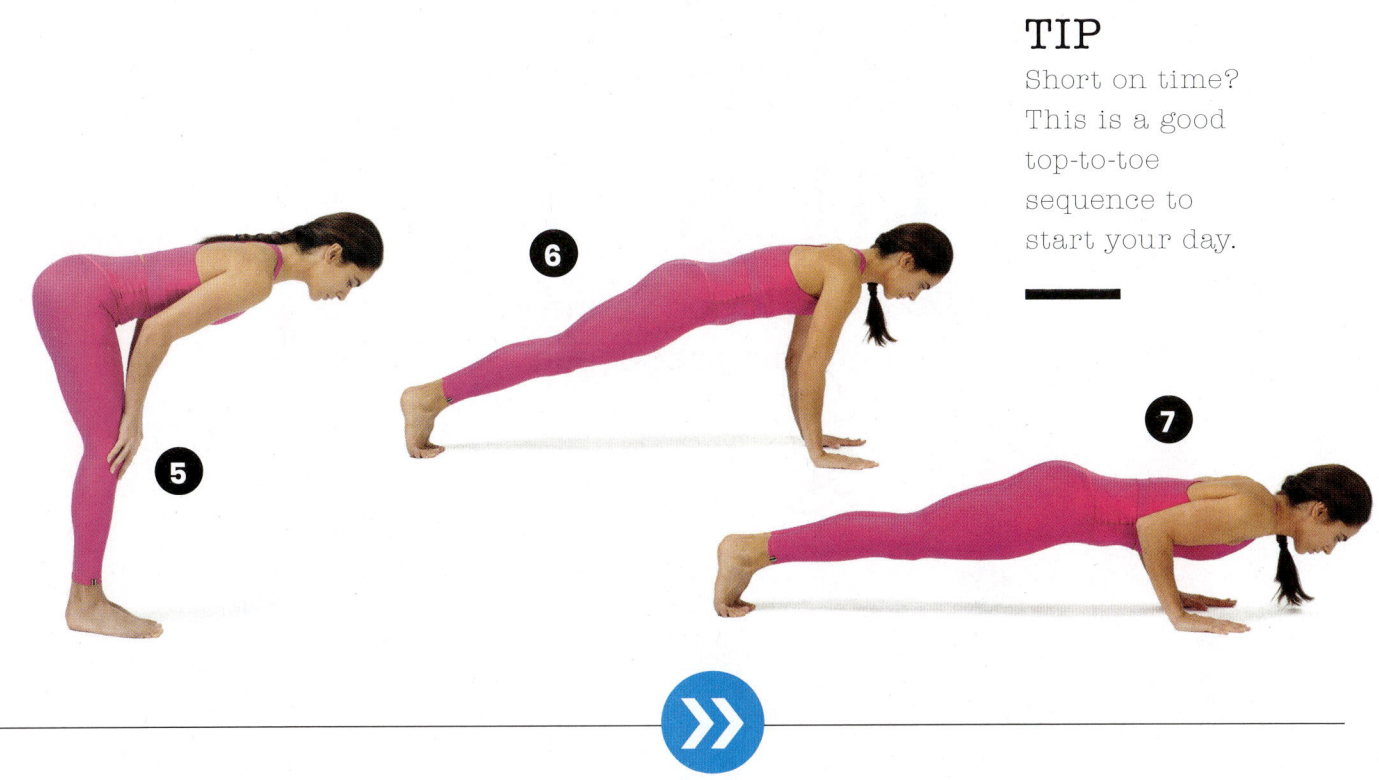

TIP
Short on time? This is a good top-to-toe sequence to start your day.

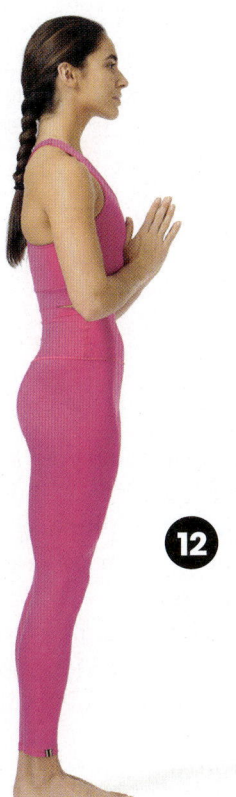

How to do it
Try practising a few rounds, gradually picking up the pace. Remember to follow your breath as always.

1. Mountain pose (p40)
Inhale into...
2. Extended mountain pose (p41)
Exhale into...
3. Chair (p44)
Inhale, straighten your legs and then exhale, bending forwards into...
4. Standing forward bend (p42)
Inhale into...
5. Half-standing forward bend (p43)
Exhale into...
6. Plank (p66)
Bend your arms and bring your body down into...
7. Four-limbed staff pose (p68)
Either bring your body onto the floor then inhale into the next move, or inhale and lift yourself straight back up into...
8. Upward-facing dog (p74)
Exhale, lifting your hips up into...
9. Downward-facing dog (p62)
Take five deep breaths here. Then inhale and step your feet forwards into...
10. Half-standing forward bend (p43)
Look up for one breath. Then exhale into...
11. Standing forward bend (p42)
Inhale your arms back up to...
12. Mountain pose (p40)

ENERGISE YOUR DAY

Wake your body and mind with this uplifting sequence

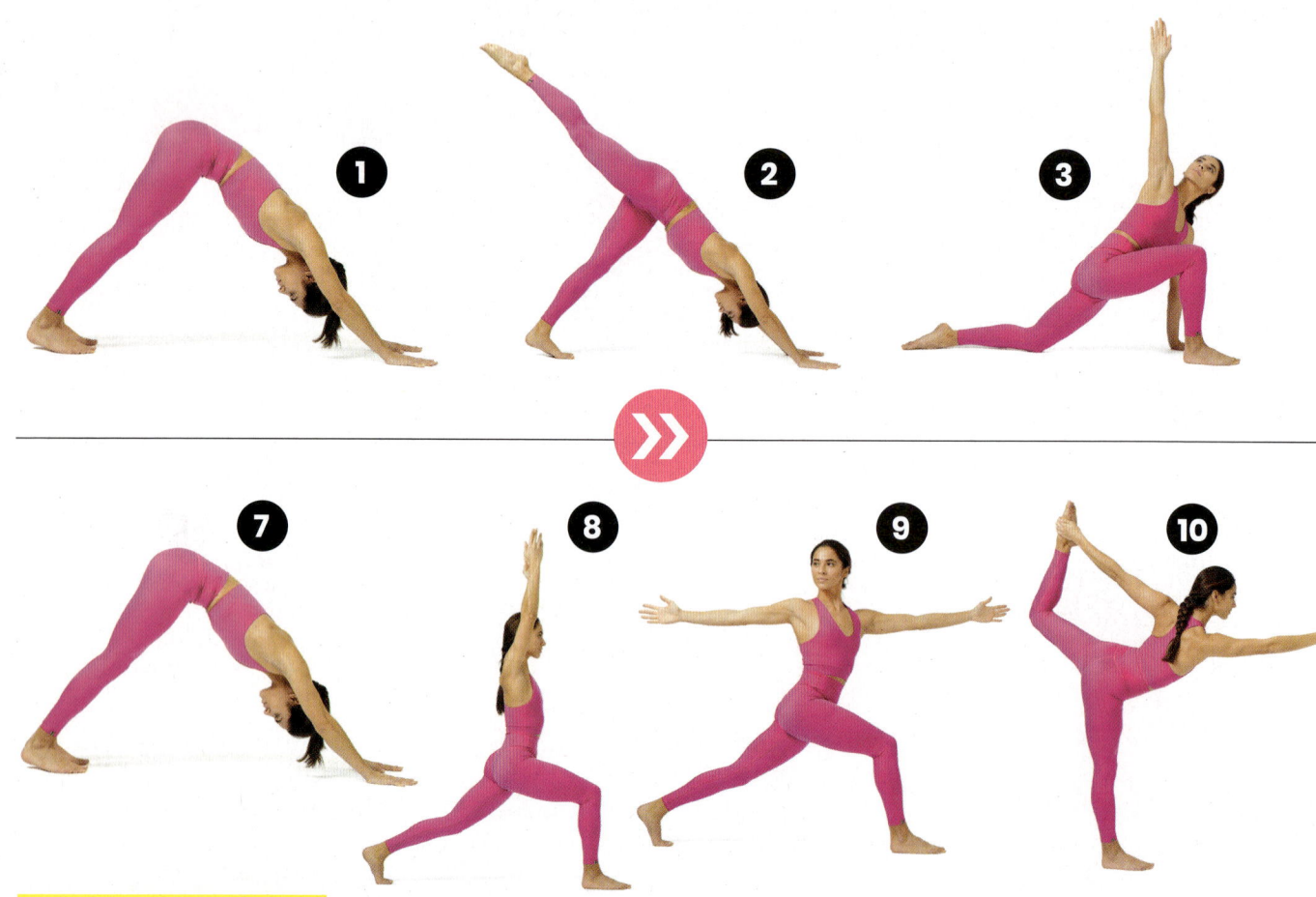

SEQUENCE

1. Downward-facing dog (p62)
Inhale and raise your right leg back into...

2. Three-limbed dog (p64)
Exhale as you step your right foot between your hands. Inhale, raise your right arm and lean your shoulder back from your ear into...

3. Lunge twist (p49)
Exhale your hands to the floor and step your right foot back into...

4. Downward-facing dog (p62)
Come down onto your knees, inhale and drop your belly towards the floor and send your chest through your arms looking up into...

5. Cow (p81)
Exhale as you round your back, pull your shoulders to your ears and tuck in your chin into...

6. Cat (p80)

Repeat steps 1-6 on your left side. Then step back into...

7. Downward-facing dog (p62)
Step your right foot forwards into...

8. High lunge (p52)
Inhale and take your arms up. Then exhale and reach your left arm forwards, your right arm back into...

9. Twisted high lunge (p53)
Inhale and reach your arms

Sequences

Morning is the ideal time to put some heart-opening poses into your yoga practice. They lift your mood, give you a natural boost of energy and enthusiasm and make space for your lungs to enable a deeper breathing pattern. When your breath is consistent and full, you're less likely to fall into the shallow or erratic breathing that accompanies a stressful state of mind.

WARM-UP
Do 3 x Sun salutation 1 and
2 x Sun salutation 2

TIP
Beginners, try taking three breaths in each pose.

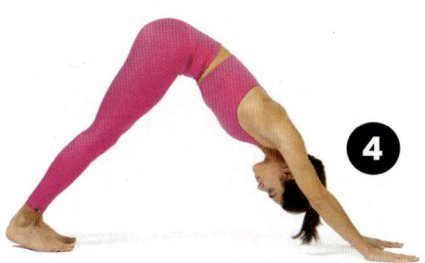
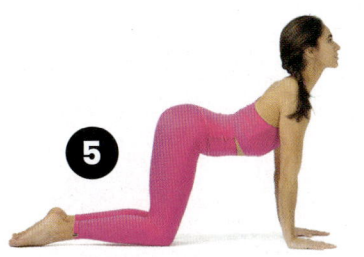
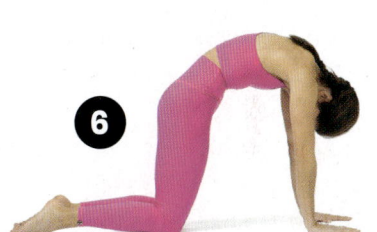

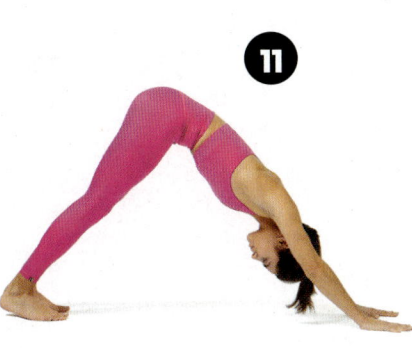
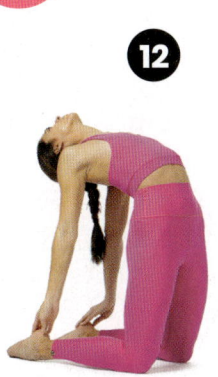
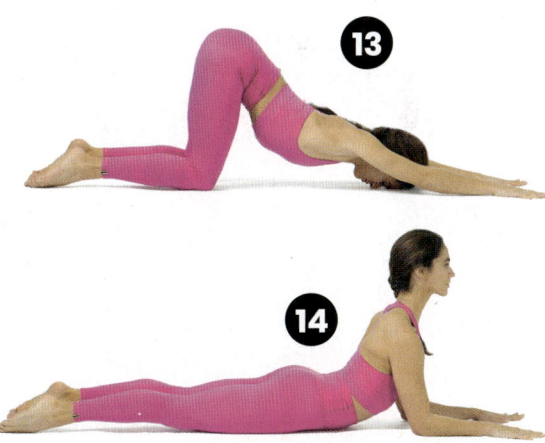

overhead, then exhale as your left hand takes your left foot in to your buttock. Inhale as you lift your ribcage forwards and upwards into...
10. Dancer (p58)
Release your leg and step back into...
11. Downward-facing dog (p62)
Repeat steps 8-10 on your left side. Then kneel down for...

12. Camel (p78)
TIP. If taking your head back causes neck strain, keep your chin tucked in. Keep your knees hip-width apart, hands on hips and hug your elbows towards each other. Relax your spine and move into...
13. Puppy dog (p100)
Keep your hips above your knees and rest your forehead

and forearms on the floor then inhale, lift your chest and slide forwards into...
14. Sphinx (p73)
Keep your fingers spread wide and press down your thigh bones and toenails as you lift up through the crown of your head. Roll onto your back for...
END Corpse pose (p92)
Rest here for five minutes.

GROUND YOURSELF

Wake your body and mind with this uplifting sequence

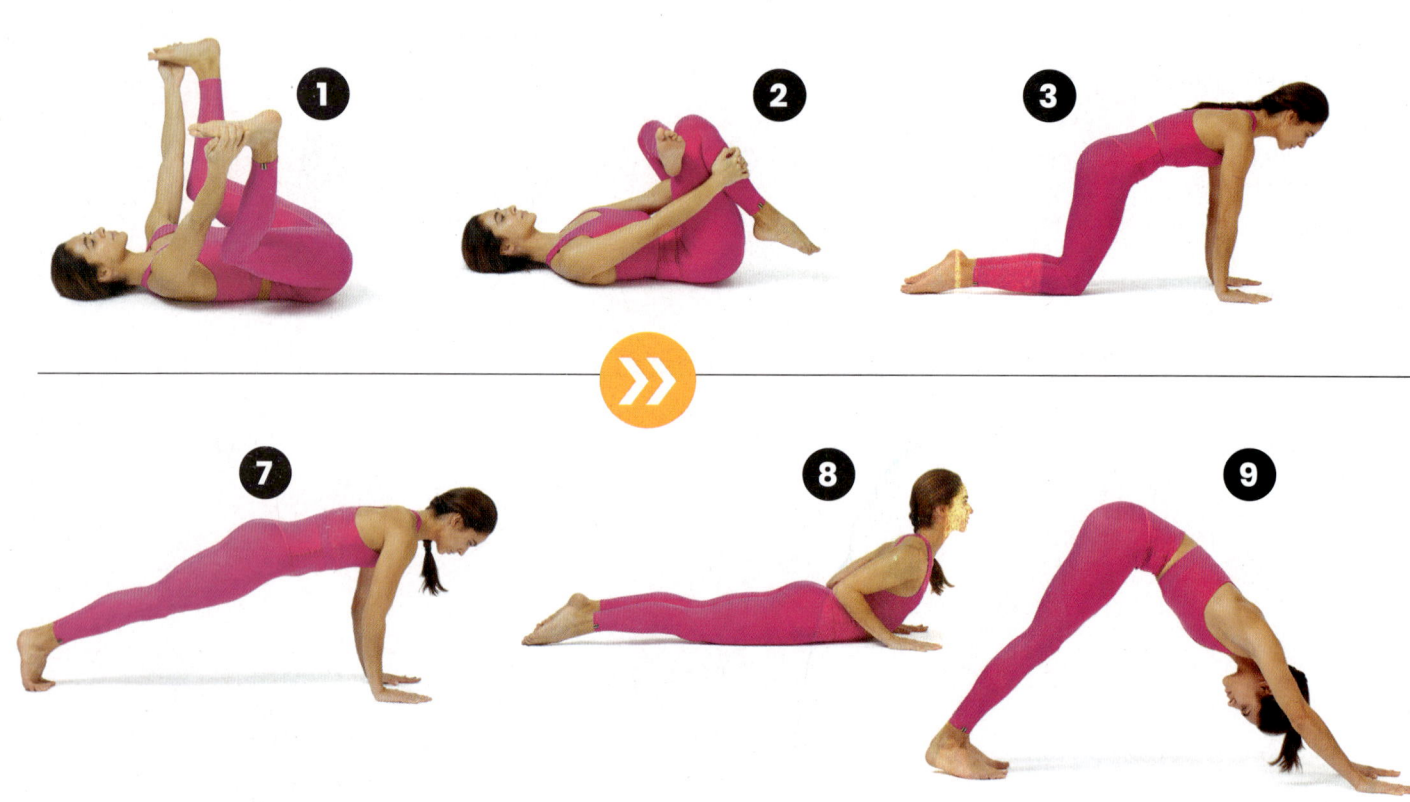

SEQUENCE

1. Happy baby (p101)
Gently rock from side to side then ground your feet hip-width apart for…

2. Eye of the needle (p101)
Do the pose on both sides, then hug your knees together, roll to one side and come up to…

3. All-fours (p100)
TIP. Try doing Lion's breath (p100) while you're in All-fours pose.
Keep your palms under your shoulders and knees hip-distance apart. Extend your right leg out to the side for…

4. Gate (p82)
Exhale back to All-fours, repeat on your left side, then inhale into…

5. Downward-facing dog (p62)
Breathe and inhale, lift your right leg high and exhale as you step your right foot to the outside of your right wrist into…

6. Lizard (p70)
Exhale and step back into…

7. Plank (p66)
Lower your belly onto the floor into…

8. Cobra (p72)
Exhale down onto your belly, place your palms

Sequences

When life is full power and you're feeling the pressure, a grounding yoga session can help let go of some of that nervous energy and slow down your brain's mental chatter. When you get stuck in 'fight or flight' mode a sequence like this – with poses that open up your hip joints and keep you close to the floor – will help encourage your system into 'rest and digest' mode.

WARM-UP

Try a seated meditation before this sequence.

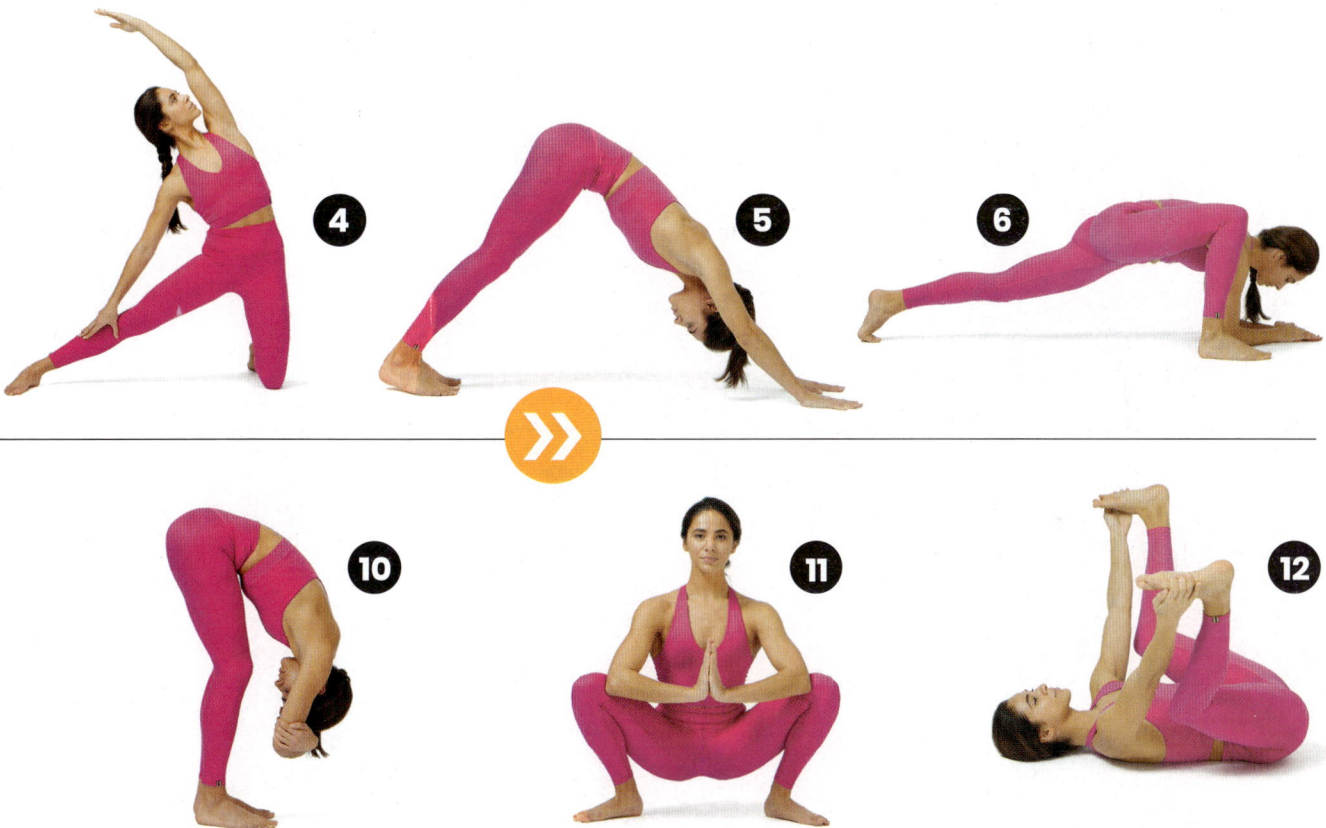

under your shoulders and inhale to...

9. Downward-facing dog (p62)
Repeat steps 6-8 on your left side. From Downward-facing dog bend your legs, look forwards, inhale and step or lightly jump your feet to your hands and exhale forwards into...

10. Rag doll pose (p42)

Walk your feet wide, turn your heels in and toes out and lower down into...

11. Garland (p60)
Roll back into...

12. Happy baby (p101)
Once you've completed the pose, recline back into...

END Corpse pose (p92)
Rest here for five minutes.

TIP
Aim to walk in nature, or a local park, today to stay feeling grounded.

FIND YOUR FOCUS

Start the day feeling sharp and focused with this centring series of moves

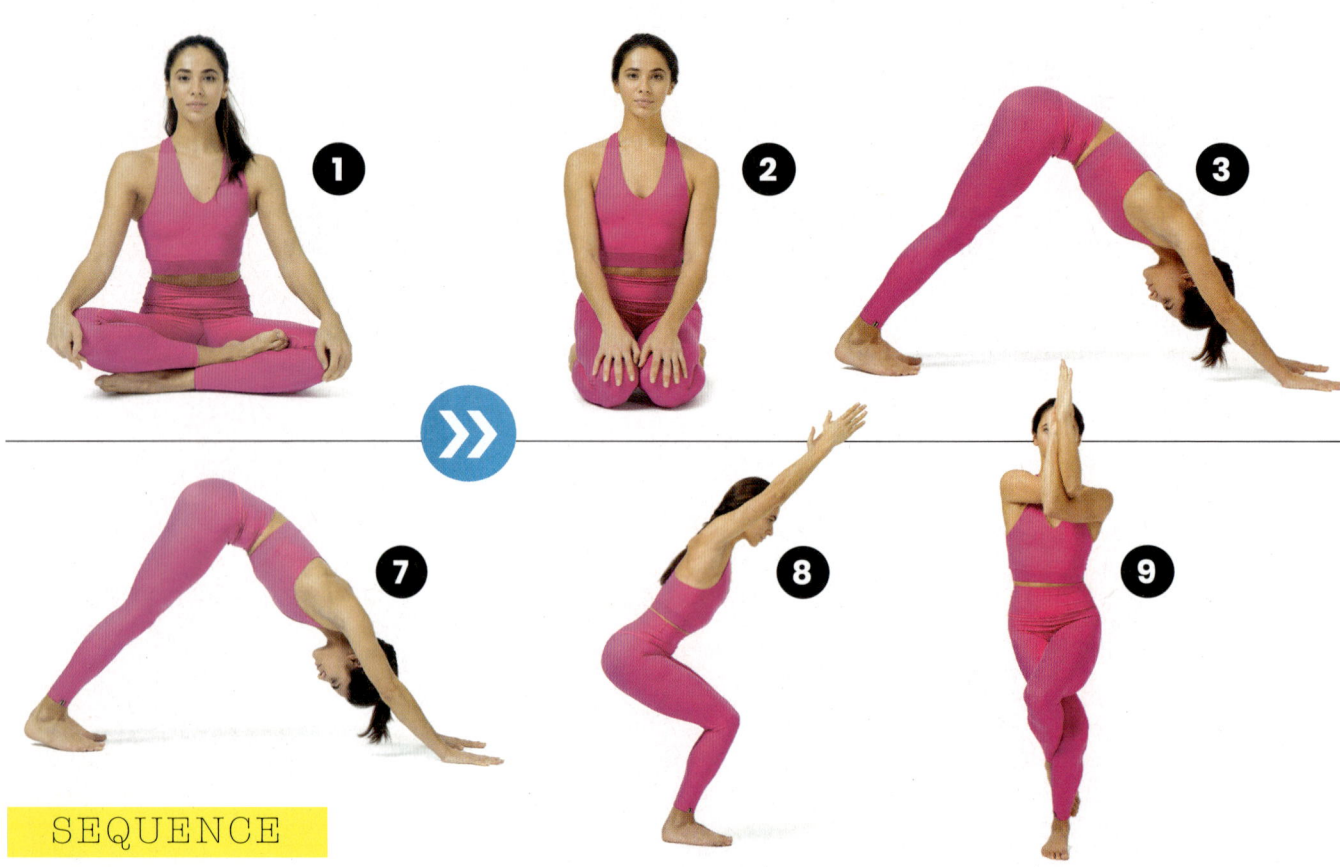

SEQUENCE

1. Easy pose (p31)
Walk your palms out in front of you, exhale deeply, then inhale back upright and switch legs. Inhale up, then exhale as you uncross your legs and move into....

TIP If you are able, cross your right thigh over your left into the legs of Cow face pose (p84).

2. Hero pose (p31)
Place your palms down on the floor in front of your knees, widen your knees, tuck your toes and lift into...

3. Downward-facing dog (p62)
Walk your hands back towards your feet, bend your legs and clasp your elbows for...

4. Rag doll pose (p42)
Gently sway your body from side to side, then inhale back up to stand in...

5. Mountain pose (p40)
Root down through your right foot, turn out your left toes and pick up your left foot to position above or below your right knee for...

6. Tree (p46)
Repeat the pose on your left side, then step down, fold forwards and walk your hands to the front of the mat for...

TIP To help your balance, find something at eye level to fix a soft gaze on.

Sequences

This sequence is perfect for the days where you need to gather your thoughts and focus on something specific – perhaps a test or a presentation or when you need clarity on a decision. The poses will help focus your mind and centre your body. They will bring you a sense of confidence and empowerment to tackle anything that comes your way with clarity and calm.

WARM-UP

A little Pranayama – or breathwork exercises (p118) – would be ideal to start your session.

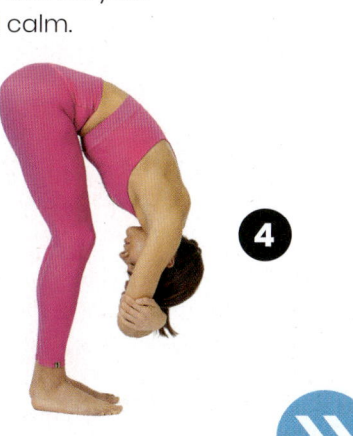
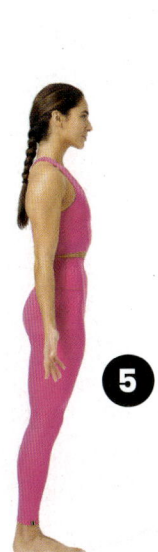
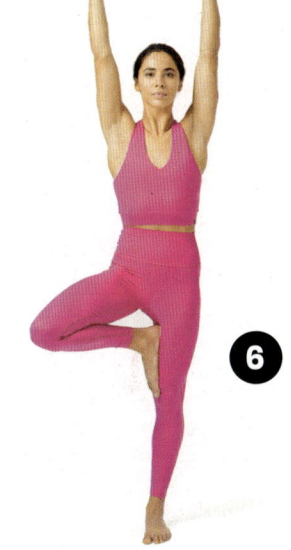

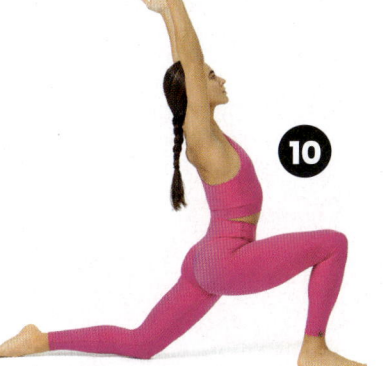
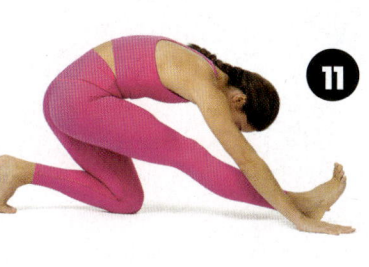
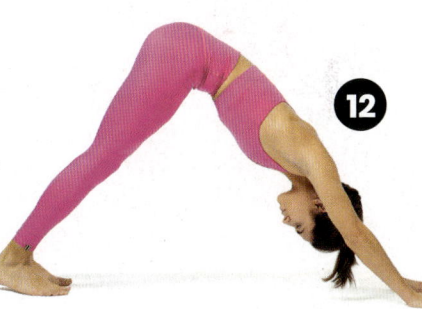

7. Downward-facing dog (p62)
Bend your legs, look forwards and inhale, step or jump your feet to your hands and fold forwards into…

8. Chair (p44)
Root down through your right foot, lift your left leg and cross it over your right leg for…

9. Eagle (p56)
If you find it hard to balance, keep your left big toe on the floor. Inhale as you unravel your arms and legs and then exhale, floating your left leg back and down into…

10. Low lunge (p48)
Ground your fingertips to frame your right foot, straighten your right leg, flex your right foot and keep your head high or bend it down towards your right knee for…

11. Half-splits (p50)
Inhale, lift your chest and straighten your back leg as you move into….

TIP Keep a cushion or yoga block handy to place under your back knee for comfort.

12. Downward-facing dog (p62)
Repeat steps 7-11 on your left side. Then, from Downward-facing dog sit down or recline for…

END Corpse pose (p92) or meditation (p122).

MORNING STRETCH

Limber up your muscles and loosen your joints with this deeply stretching sequence

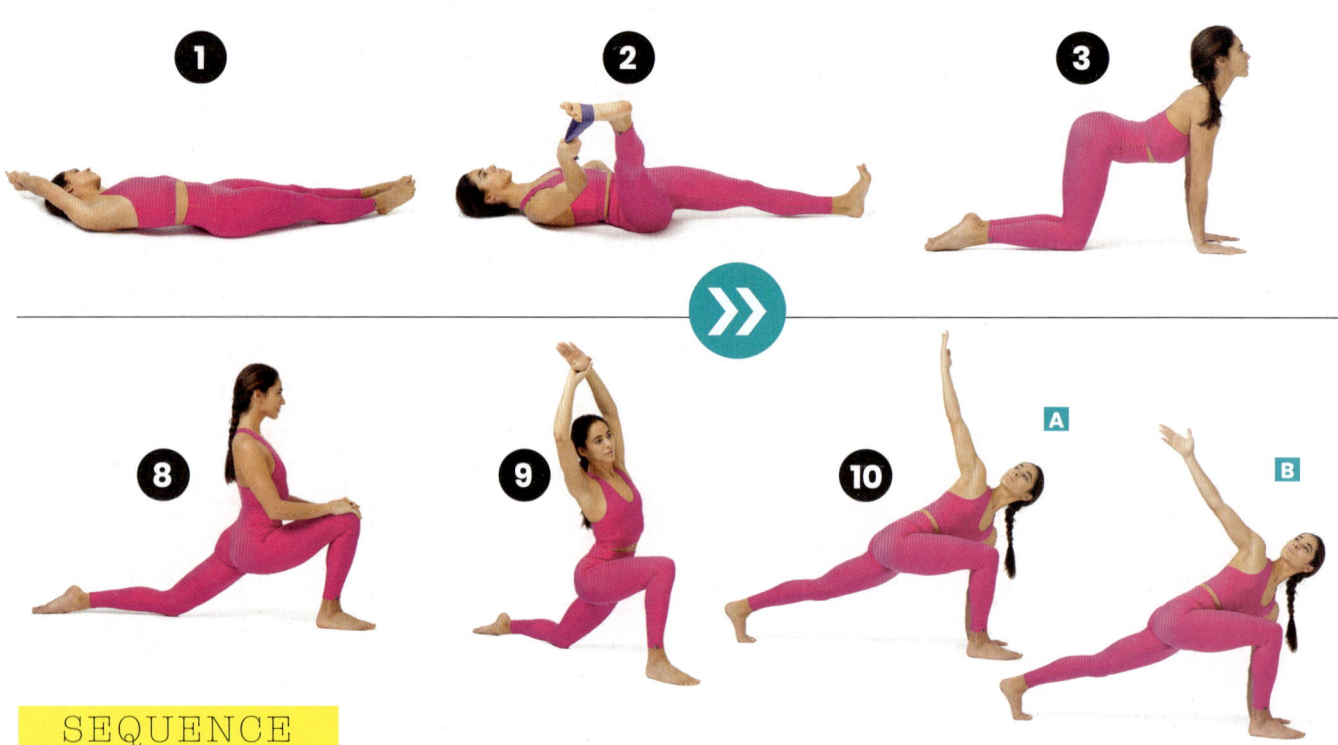

SEQUENCE

1. Banana pose (p88)
Stretch on your right side by clasping your right wrist over your head at the back left corner of your mat and feet at the front left corner, then change sides. Reach for your strap and make a stirrup around your right foot for...

2. Reclining hand-to-big-toe (p90)
Repeat on your left leg, then lower your leg, hug your knees into your chest, roll to one side and move onto all-fours for...

3. Cow (p81)
Inhale and then exhale into...

4. Cat (p80)
Relax your spine, tuck your toes and move into...

5. Downward-facing dog (p62)
For a shoulder stretch, reach your right hand back to clasp your left outer ankle or shin into...

6. Revolved downward dog (p63)
Repeat on your left side then inhale and raise your right leg into...

7. 3-limbed downward dog (p64)
Bend your right leg, reach back with your right knee and circle your ankle. Straighten your leg, square your hips and step your right foot to the inside of your right wrist for...

8. Low lunge (p48)
Place your right hand on right knee to keep your hips level, then inhale, raise your arms high and catch your left wrist as you lean your body to the right into...

Sequences

Sometimes the body feels as if it really doesn't want to move in the mornings, especially in the winter months. Ease into your day gently with an emphasis on stretching to open up slowly. If you have time, spend longer in each pose than you usually would and notice if that helps. Keep a yoga strap close by – or improvise with a belt or scarf.

WARM-UP

Begin by relaxing in Corpse pose (p92).

TIP
Hold Corpse pose (p92) for longer than usual. Have a blanket handy.

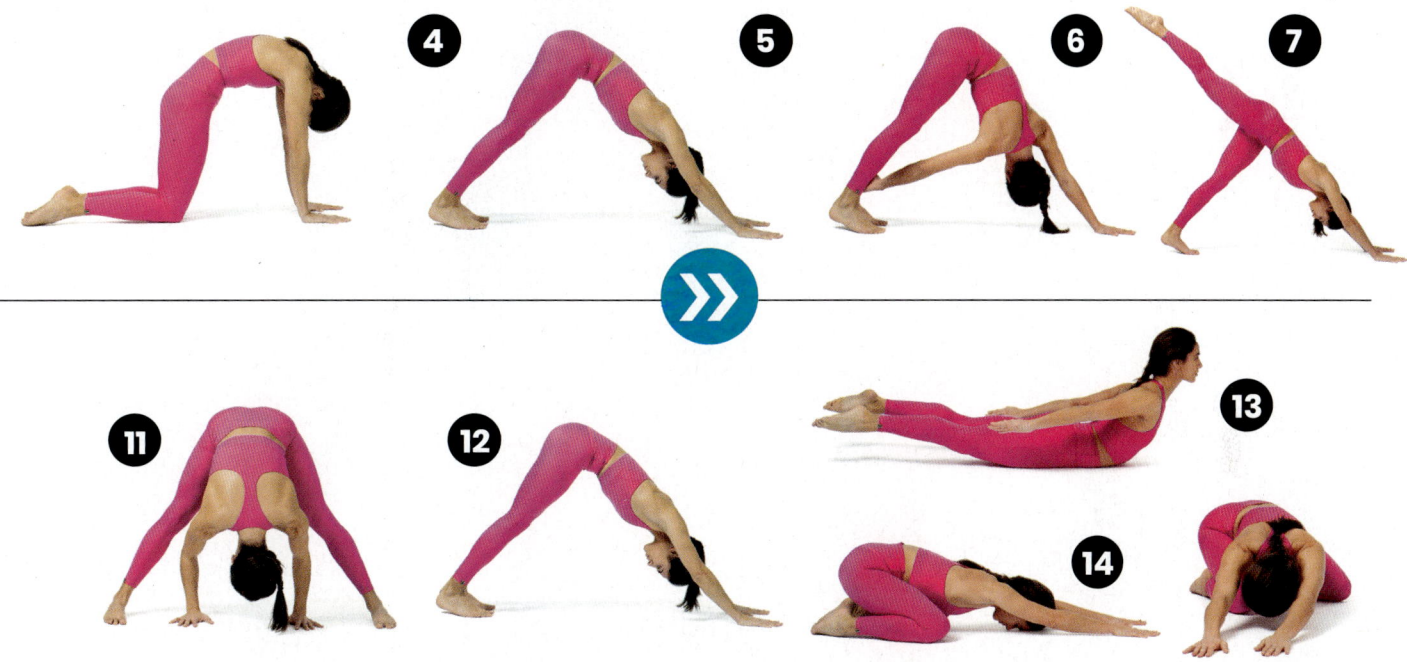

9. Low lunge stretch (p49) Release your left hand to the floor and straighten your back leg as you inhale into…

10 (A). Lunge twist (p49) Make big, slow sweeping circles with your right hand to open up your shoulder joint. **10 (B).** Then exhale, place your right hand next to the left and make a quarter turn to your left for…

11. Wide-legged forward bend (p54) Either keep your palms grounded below your shoulders or clasp your hands together behind you and lift your arms overhead. Bend your legs and come onto your fingertips as you lift your chest and turn towards to your right foot. Frame it with your hands and step back into…

12. Downward-facing dog (p62) *Repeat steps 5-10 on the left side.* After circling your left arm, step back into Downward-facing dog. Lower down onto your tummy and reach your arms back behind you for…

13. Locust (p76) Rest then repeat x2. Lower your limbs, place your palms under your shoulders and press up to all-fours and back into…

14. Extended child's pose (p87) Stretch your hands in front of you and walk them to the right and then the left. Then recline into…

END Corpse pose (p92) or meditation (p122)

115

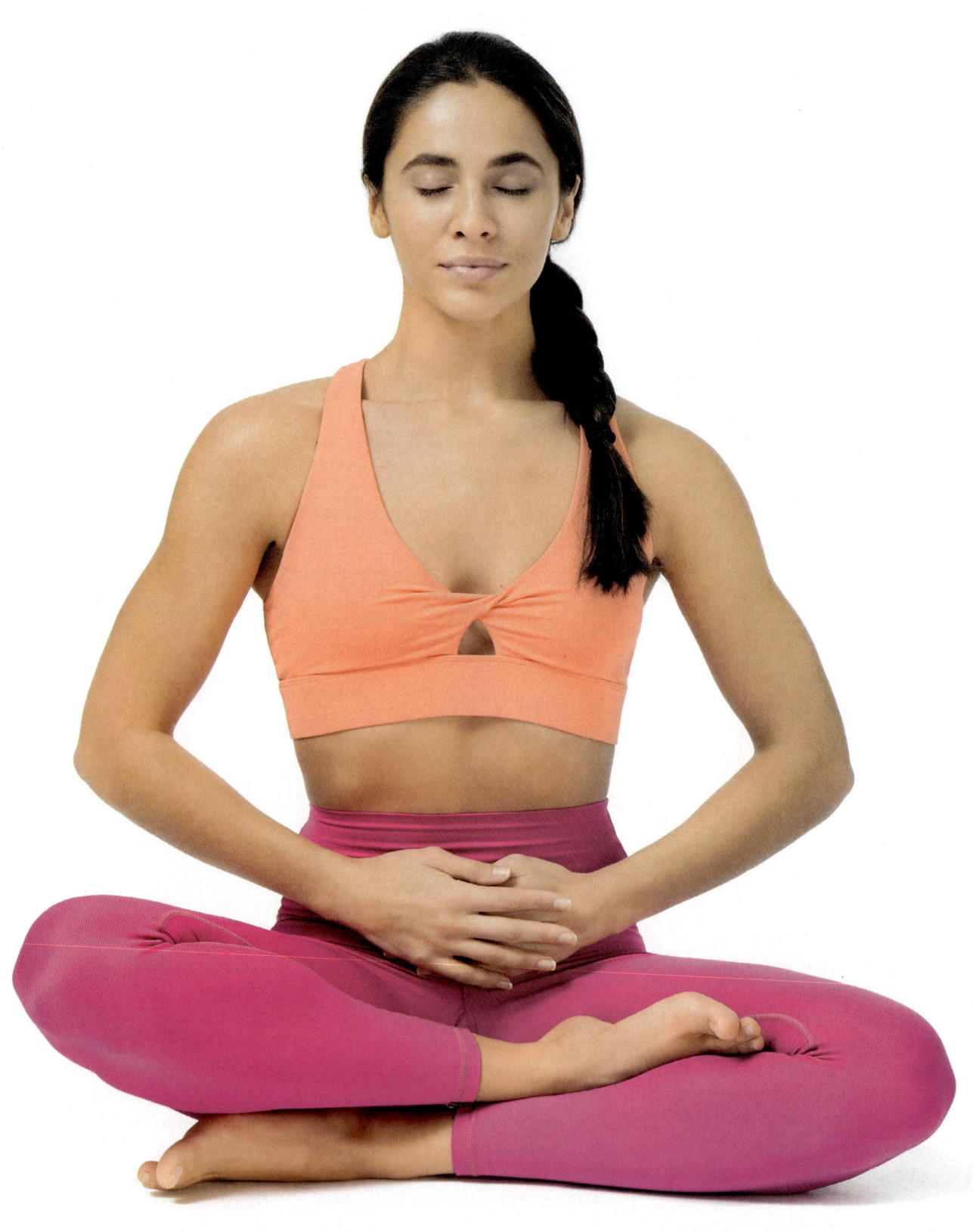

// TAKE IT FURTHER

Hopefully, you're already enjoying the benefits of your morning yoga practice. Now, it's time to take it further and deepen the mind and body rewards by adding some yogic breathing and meditation exercises. From energising your body and boosting your mood to focusing your brain and creating a feeling of calm, in this section, you'll find a variety of quick and easy exercises. Mix and match them with your yoga sequences to suit your daily goals.

Breathe INTO BEING

Deepen your yoga practice and boost your wellbeing by adding simple, yogic breathing exercises to your morning sessions from breathwork expert Hanna-Jade Browne

"Including a regular breathing practice as part of your morning routine is one of the easiest and most effective tools to improve your wellbeing and physical health.

Just as the physical body has veins, arteries and nerves which deliver and receive vital fluids and signals to and from its organs, there is a subtle energetic system of channels known as 'nadis' which carry and receive vital life force energy, also known as 'prana'. For optimum wellbeing, this energy needs to be in motion. However, emotions can block the natural flow of energy through the nadis. If an emotion becomes stuck, it can stagnate and become pathological. In breathwork practice, the nadis are charged, opened and purified so prana can flow freely.

There are many methods of yogic breath control (Pranayama) and breathing exercises, all with different benefits – some are calming, others more stimulating. How you feel in the morning will determine which exercise you choose to use.

In general, it's recommended to practise five to 15 minutes of Pranamaya and breathwork each morning. If you follow a morning meditation and/or yoga practice, it's best to do your breathwork first as it will prepare your mind and body for a deeper and more connected practice.

At first, it may feel uncomfortable or awkward, but like anything new, give it some time and soon it will become second nature and even quite blissful."

Breathwork

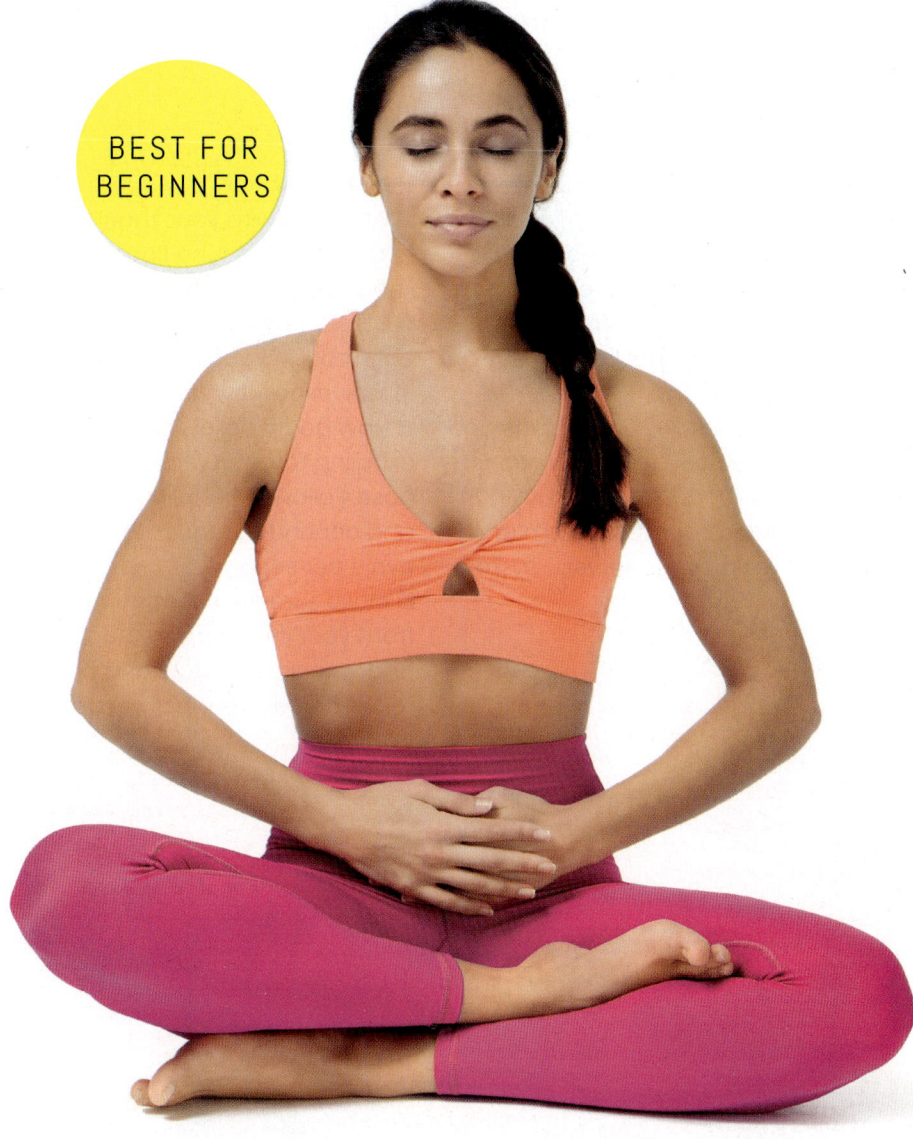

BEST FOR BEGINNERS

Breathwork tips

Here are some useful tips to keep in mind:

- Make sure you're in a quiet space, free of distractions.
- Avoid straining — if you feel dizzy or experience any discomfort, stop for a moment and sit quietly until you feel better.
- If you feel anxious, stop the exercise and rest until the sensation passes.
- Try a vigorous breath first (such as Bhastrika, p120), followed by a calming technique (such as Cardiac Coherence Breathing, p121).
- Start off slowly. Perhaps perform a one-minute exercise for the first week to allow your body to adjust. Then work up to five or 15 minutes — listen to your body.

DIAPHRAGMATIC OR BELLY BREATHING

Here is an easy exercise to get you started. There are many benefits for learning how to breathe deeply. As a yoga practitioner, deep breathing can help improve your posture, gently stretch and tone your core muscles (including your pelvic floor), stimulate the relaxation response and increase mental clarity.

How to do it

- Sit in a comfortable position with your spine supported or comfortably straight, or lie down on your back.
- Place both your hands on your lower belly and relax your abdominal muscles.
- Slowly inhale through your nose for four counts, drawing the air down into the lower lobes of your lungs, noticing your abdomen expanding.
- On the same inhale, feel your ribcage expand outwards as your breath enters upwards and sense your chest expanding slightly.
- Pause for a moment, then exhale out of your mouth as if you're sighing.
- At the end of the exhalation, gently draw your belly button towards your spine, releasing any residual air out of the bottom of your lungs.
- Pause for a moment and allow the vacuum in your lungs to draw your next breath in.

BEST FOR ENERGY

BHASTRIKA, OR BELLOWS BREATH

The next time you wake up feeling tired, instead of reaching for a cup of coffee, try this energetic breathing practice instead. The benefits are instant, offering an increase in energy, clarity and focus due to the release of mood-boosting endorphins and increased oxygen absorption in the blood, as well as kick-starting your metabolism and regulating your nervous system.

How to do it
- Sit up tall with your shoulders relaxed, or lie on the floor with your knees bent and hip-width apart.
- Take a few, deep breaths in and out through your nose. With each inhale, expand your lower belly fully.
- Now begin bellows breathing by exhaling forcefully through your nose. Follow by inhaling forcefully and continue at the rate of one cycle per second.
- Make sure your breath is coming from your diaphragm. Keep your head, neck, shoulders and chest relaxed while your belly expands in and out.

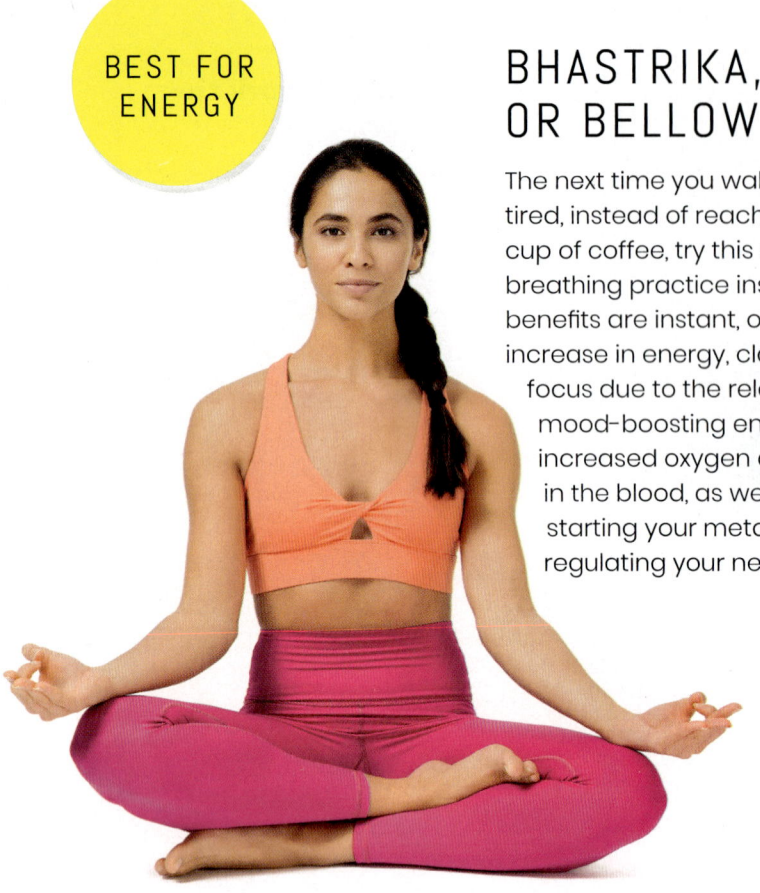

BEST FOR MINDFULNESS

ANAPANASATI

It's believed that the Anapanasati breathing technique was created by the Buddha himself. The initial practice is simple, its purpose is for you to feel the sensations created by the movements of your breath in your body. Practising this exercise increases your sense of mindfulness, breath and body awareness. It aids emotional clearing, calms your limbic system and prepares you for a deeper state of meditation.

How to do it
- Sit or lie down in stillness with your eyes closed. Observe the natural flow of your breath.
- To keep your mind focused, count your inhales and exhales from one to 10 and/or tune into the sensation of your breath expanding and releasing in your belly. More advanced mindfulness practitioners can observe the sensation of the breath at the tip of your nose and top of your upper lip.
- Make sure that your breathing is neutral, soft and equal.
- Practise Anapanasati for as long as you like.

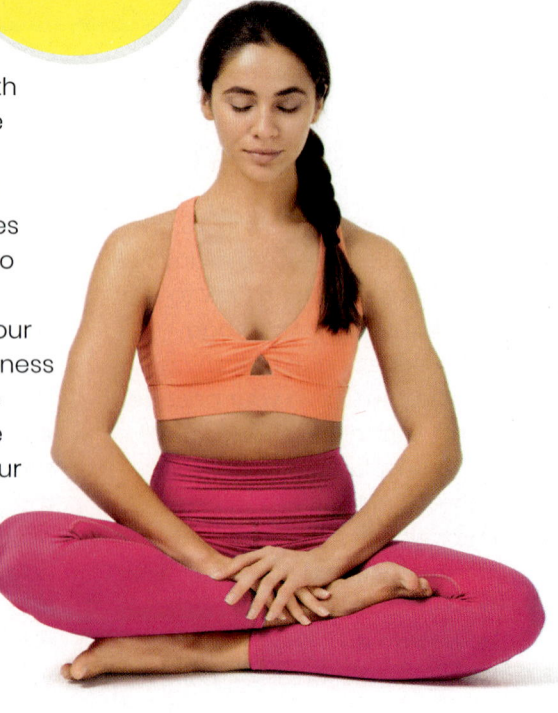

Breathwork

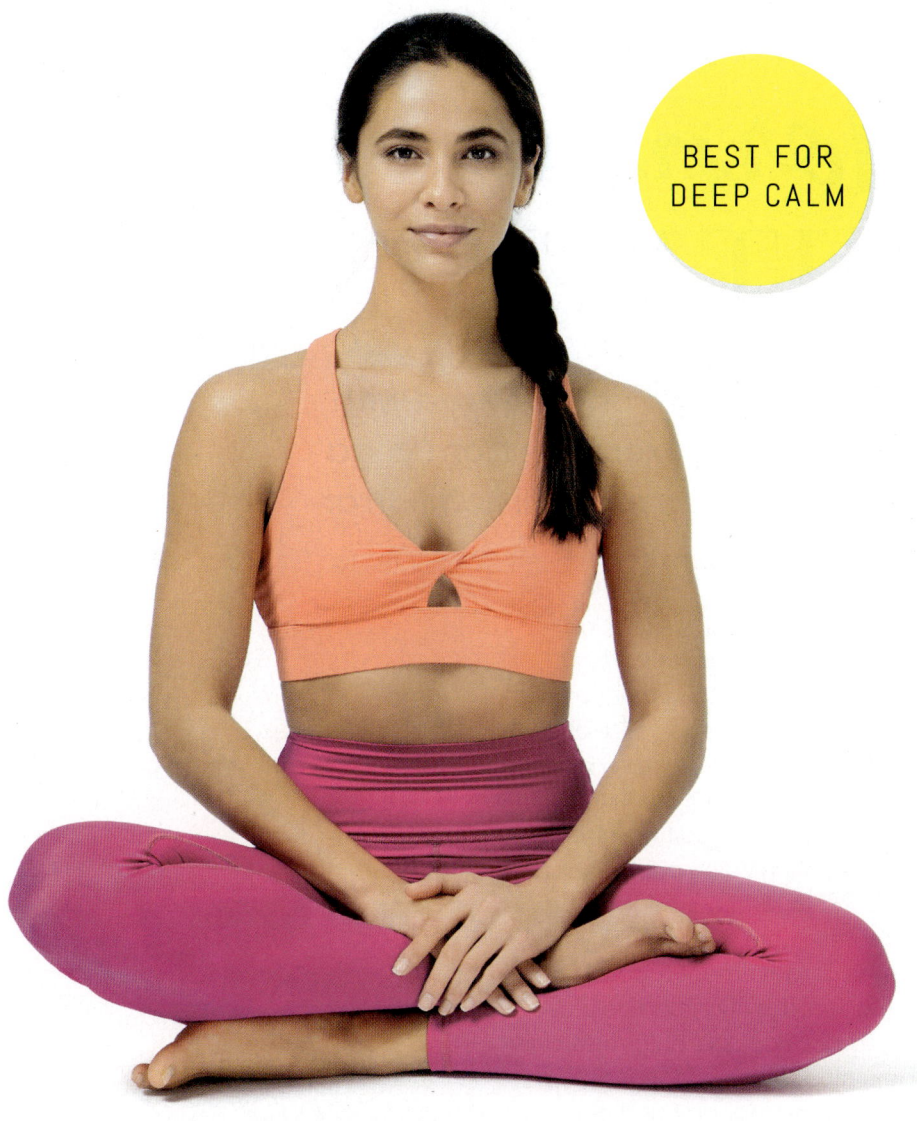

BEST FOR DEEP CALM

CARDIAC COHERENCE BREATHING

Rhythmic breathing causes your body/mind to sync into a cardiac coherence state, where your heart, mind and body fall into the same rhythm. Sometimes called 'The Zone', it's a state where you feel connected to your deepest self, to others and to life itself. Heart coherence occurs when your breathing and heart rhythm become synchronised and operate at the same frequency. Practising this technique is good for your heart, mind and soul. Your blood pressure falls, your emotions become calm, and your thoughts disappear.

How to do it
- Relax and find a comfortable position to breathe, which will be supportive in keeping you calm but attentive.
- Inhale into your belly for five seconds.
- Exhale for another five seconds.
- Repeat for three to five minutes.
- Allow your thoughts to come and go; notice if you become distracted and return to counting your breaths.
- Allow your body/mind the space to unwind and come into coherence. The key is to be patient and trust your breath.

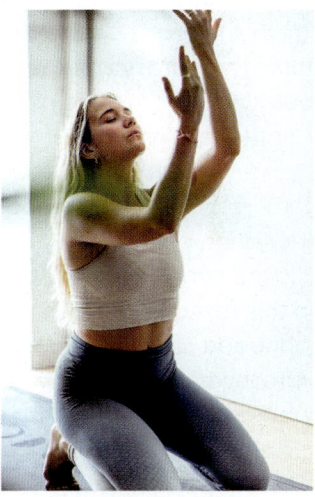

Meet your instructor
Hanna-Jade Browne is a qualified yoga and breathwork teacher, and founder of Embodhi Breath. She is a therapeutic practitioner in integrative breathwork and qualified with schools worldwide including Rebirthing, Transformational Breath and Bio-dynamic Breathwork & Trauma Release System, as well as in sound healing with the Acutonics system and Reiki to a master level.
For Hanna-Jade's full biography, turn to page 130.

Morning MEDITATION

Start your day feeling calm and centred with some simple meditation exercises from yoga teacher and mindfulness expert Ali Roff Farrar

Q What are the benefits of morning meditation?
A. 'Meditation is fantastic for your health – for example, people who meditate have 76 per cent fewer days off work due to illness compared with those who don't meditate. Meditating activates the parasympathetic nervous system – moving us from "fight, flight or freeze" mode (where many of us spend our time!) to "rest and digest" mode. So meditation can be really beneficial to ensure we start our day in this rest and digest mode, with our heart rate and blood pressure lowered in the physical body, and stress, anxiety and tension lowered in the emotional body. Morning meditation, in particular, can set us up for a productive day; reducing our reliance on caffeine, increasing our ability to multi-task, and creating a more positive mindset.'

Q Is meditation a good partner for yoga?
A. 'Definitely. Traditionally, the physical postures (asanas) of yoga are used to make the body strong and comfortable so we can meditate free from distraction in our bodies. But yoga is also movement meditation. I don't beat myself up if I don't have time for both in a busy day, because for me, meditation and yoga are one. But they can support each other too. We may find it easier to meditate after a yoga session when our bodies feel blissed out, and our minds have become more still through yogic physical movement meditation. Equally, meditation can help us feel grounded and balanced, and be a nice transition for the mind between a busy day and our physical yoga practice.'

Q Is it ok to just do a short meditation when you're busy?
A. 'Of course! There's no "right" way to meditate, and it's better to do just a few mindful breaths each day, than believe the only way to meditate properly is by sitting cross-legged in silence for an hour at a time, something many of us would only be able to achieve once a month! A really easy meditation you can do anywhere, is a Mindful breath meditation (p125) – the breath is with you always, everywhere you go, so it's a great tool to meditate with.'

Ali's morning meditation practice

" I usually meditate in the morning. It might just be a few rounds of deep breathing if I'm short on time — box breath is my favourite (breathe in to the count of four, hold for four, breathe out for four, hold for four, and repeat). I also like to do a dedicated morning practice, either in bed or on my yoga mat, before I begin physical practice, such as a gratitude meditation which is a grounding way to begin the day, or an 'Om Shanti Om' mantra meditation which means 'I radiate peace'. I visualise the sun rising and light surrounding me and radiating from me. I also love to do a shower meditation — as I run the water I check in with my body, my heart and my mind and ask 'what is here today?' Whatever meditation I choose, I feel I start my day more consciously. Taking the time to check in with yourself before you give any time, attention or energy to anyone or anything else, is one of the greatest acts of self-love there is. "

Meditation

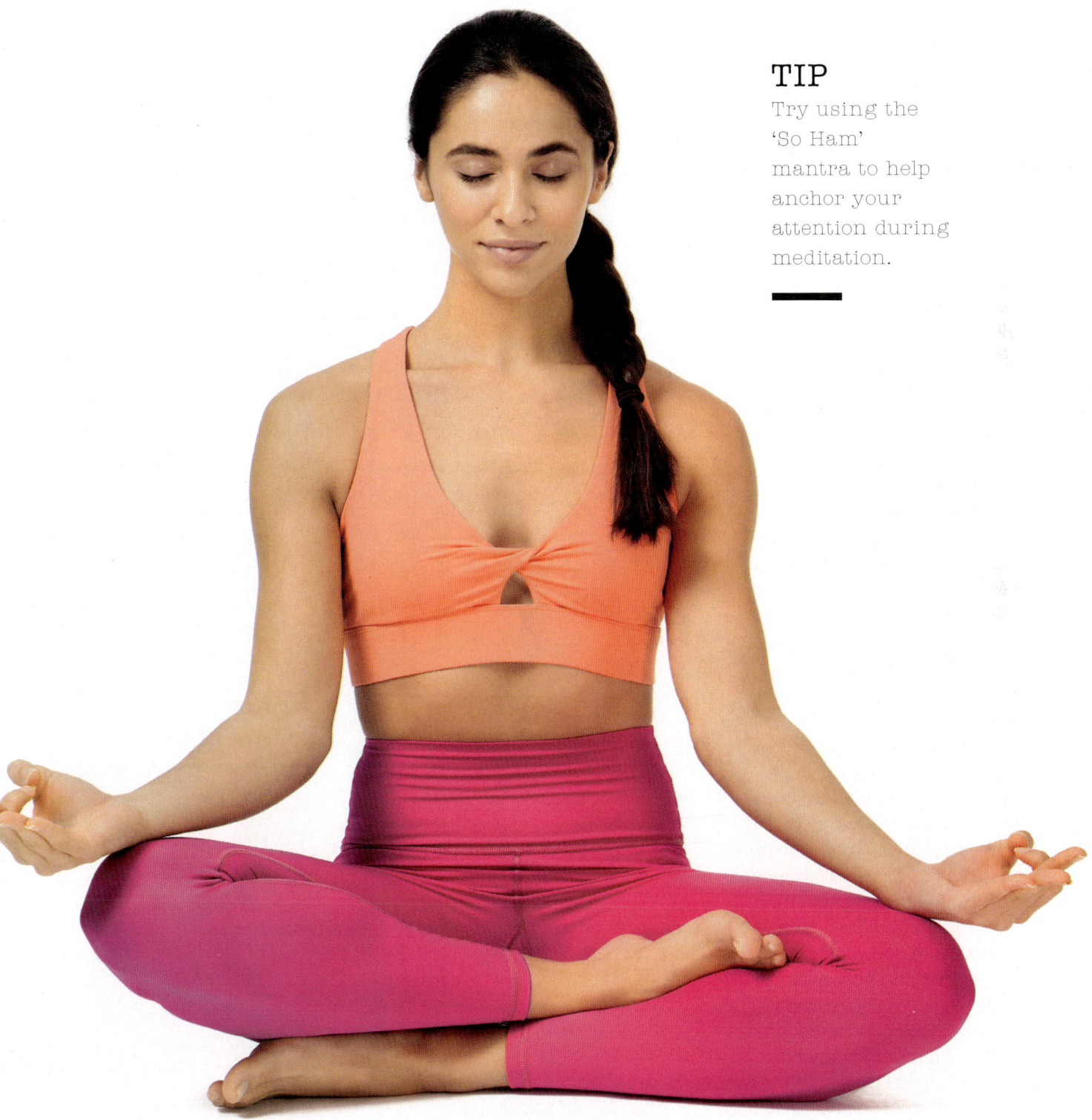

TIP
Try using the 'So Ham' mantra to help anchor your attention during meditation.

MINDFUL MOVEMENT
MEDITATION

Moving the body with the breath can be a wonderful meditation practice for those who find it difficult to sit still. Try this Mindful movement meditation which helps to still your mind, and calm your breath and your body.

- Stand in stillness for a few breaths, just taking a minute to arrive in the moment; feel the ground beneath your feet and observe your breath.
- Bring your hands up to your chest, palms facing outwards.
- On your next exhale, slowly push your arms away, as if you are pushing a ball of energy away from your body.
- At the end of your exhale, with your arms fully extended, turn your palms to face your body.
- Inhale, and draw your hands back towards your chest, as if you are gathering energy and pulling it back in towards your body.
- Continue to inhale and exhale with this arm movement, pushing energy away with your exhale and back in with your inhale.
- Keep your mind focused on your breath and your body. If a thought creeps into your mind to distract you, that's ok. Just notice the thought and let it go, then draw your attention back to your breath and your body.
- Continue this slow, mindful movement for a few minutes, allowing your mind to become quiet and your movements to become fluid. Come to stillness once again at the end, observing how you feel.

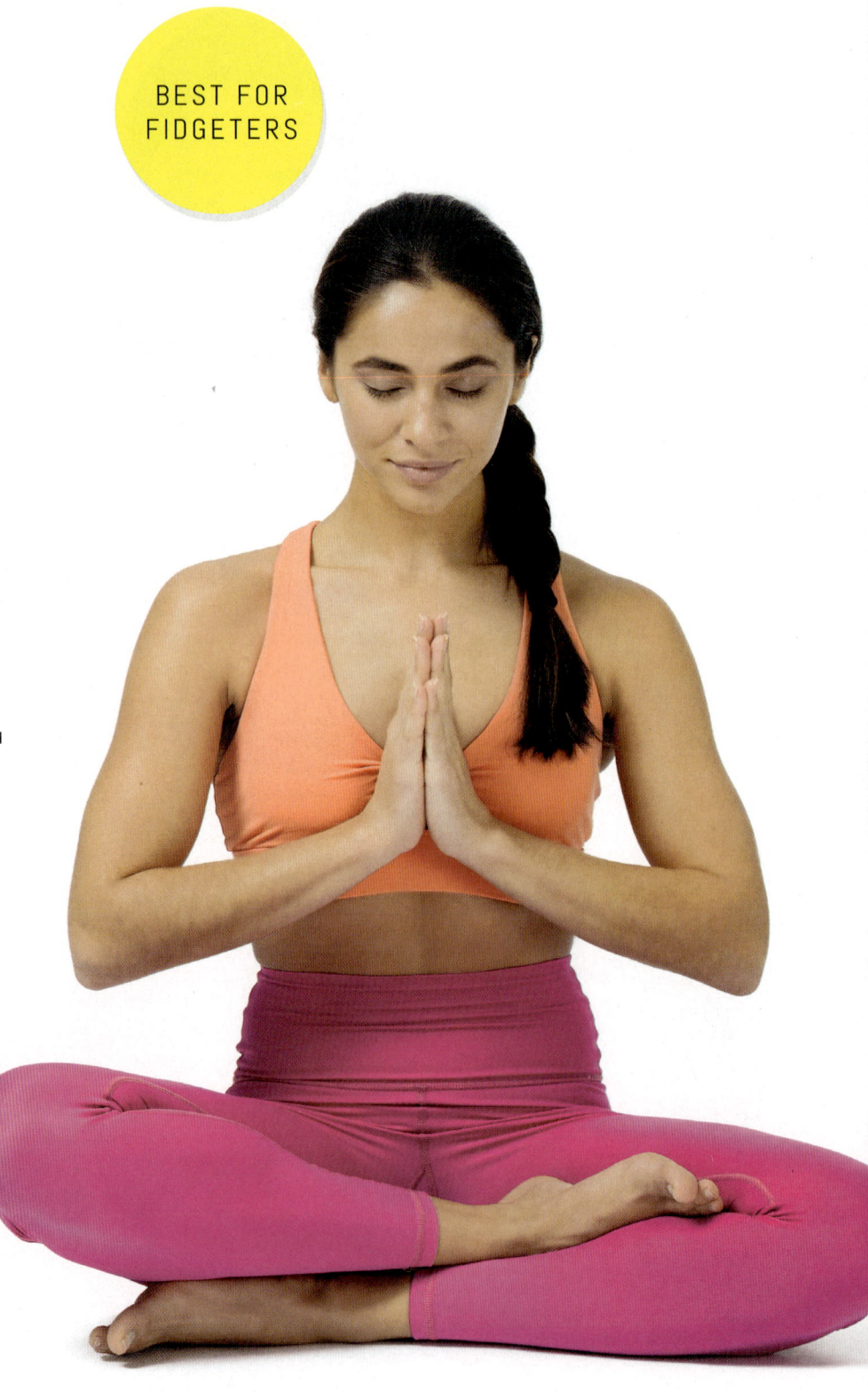

BEST FOR FIDGETERS

Meditation

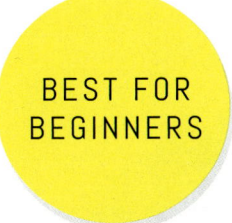

BEST FOR BEGINNERS

BEST FOR FOCUS

MINDFUL BREATH
MEDITATION

This simple meditation is a powerful way to slow down your mind and your breath, signalling to your body that you're safe and well, moving you into the 'rest and digest' parasympathetic nervous system. Practise the meditation for between two and 10 minutes to feel its soothing benefits.

■ Sit or lie quietly and place your awareness gently onto your breath, like a butterfly resting on a flower.
■ Observe your breath – watch it come in and out, as you inhale and exhale.
■ Where does your breath enter your body? What does it feel like? What is the quality of your breath? Where do you feel your breath expand in your body? What does it sound like?
■ Be curious about every quality, every aspect, as you follow your breath with your awareness.
■ If a thought comes along and distracts you from your breath, that's fine – the mind's job is to think, just like the heart's job is to beat. Simply notice the thought, let it go and come back to your breath.

INNER CONNECTION 'SO HAM'
MEDITATION

Using a mantra can be a wonderful, meaningful anchor for your focus in meditation. Try this mantra for cultivating inner connection, building up to between five to 30 minutes.

■ Find a quiet place to sit in stillness, propping your sitting bones up onto a rolled-up blanket or cushion to tilt your pelvis for a comfortable seat. Close your eyes and rest your hands on your thighs, palms facing upwards towards the sky.
■ Introduce yourself to the mantra 'So Ham' – meaning 'I am' in Sanskrit. This mantra allows you to connect to yourself rather than your thoughts, therefore connecting you to the 'ultimate reality' (rather than the mental chatter in your head). It also helps you to identify yourself with the universe or something greater than you.
■ Using the mantra 'So Ham', begin to say the words in your mind, linking their intention to the meaning above.
■ Now begin to link your breath to the mantra – in your mind say 'So' (I) on the inhale, and 'Ham' (am) on the exhale, continuing in this way.
■ Keep your awareness intently focused on the mantra and on these words, gradually focusing inwards and deeper, to settle on the still awareness in the background of your mind.

> *" It only takes a few breaths to become more conscious, more aware of how you are that day "*

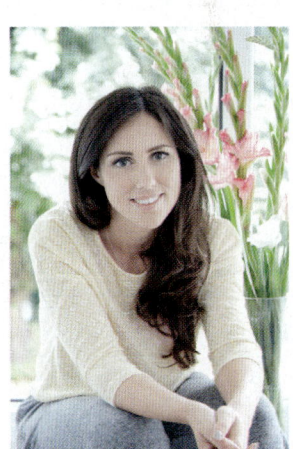

Meet your instructor

Ali Roff Farrar is a yoga teacher, mindfulness expert, wellness editor, author, and Wellness Director at **Psychologies** magazine. Her debut book **The Wellfulness Project** (Aster) is out now.

EMBRACE THE DAY

Stay happy and healthy by adding some simple yogic rituals into your morning

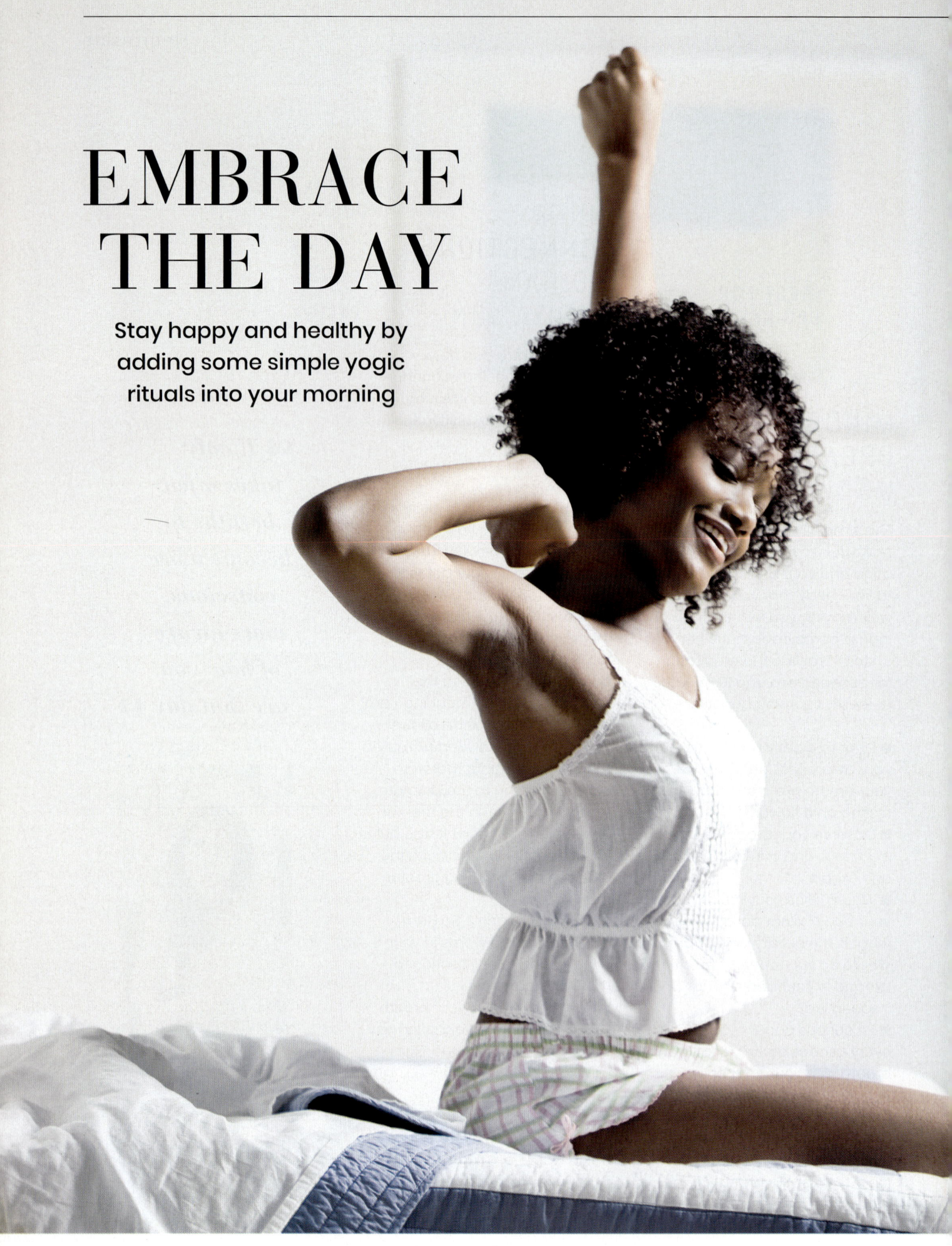

Morning rituals

Have you ever had that 'jet lagged' feeling after staying up late watching TV or sleeping through your alarm? The 24/7 nature of modern life means our natural bodyclock or circadian rhythms can become disrupted, leading to fatigue, depression and potential ill health. The good news is, introducing some simple yogic rituals (known in Ayurvedic philosophy as dinacharya) into your day, can reconnect you with your bodyclock and help you find your flow again. As simple as taking a morning shower or practising meditation, here are the changes you can make today.

> **"** *Practising gratitude in your waking moments can turn your mornings around* **"**

1 Wake up early

Have you noticed that the later you wake up in the morning, the more sleepy and sluggish you feel? According to Ayurvedic philosophy, this is because mornings are characterised by the kapha state, meaning your body feels slow and heavy. To counteract kapha's influence, it's best to wake as early as possible and do stimulating activities such as exercise or lively mental tasks. Ayurvedic physicians and yogis recommend waking at sunrise. At first, you'll probably need to set your alarm to do this but eventually, your body will learn to wake naturally with the daylight. Give it a try tomorrow, you'll be surprised how good you feel!

2 Be grateful

It's natural to feel a bit grouchy when you first wake up, especially if you're not a morning person. But research shows that making a conscious effort to foster a sense of gratitude in your waking moments can turn your mornings around, flooding your mind with positive thoughts and removing the negative emotions we often carry with us into our working day. Every morning when you wake, jot down three things you feel grateful for that day, however small. For example, it could be gratitude for your home, for cuddles with your pet, the prospect of breakfast or the sunlight shining through your window. Don't worry if doing this feels unnatural or repetitive. Persevere and you'll be amazed the difference it makes to your life.

> *"It's best to leave two hours between eating a meal and doing yoga so stick to warm water and lemon or herbal tea before your practice"*

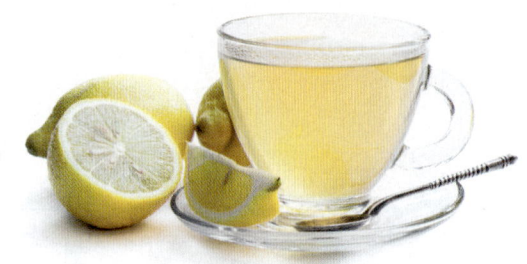

3 Freshen up

Probably the first thing you do after eating breakfast or before leaving the house is clean your teeth. But, according to Ayurvedic medicine, the best time to cleanse your mouth is before you eat in the morning. A combination of oil pulling (swilling coconut or sesame oil around your mouth for 10 minutes before spitting it out), tongue scraping (cleaning your tongue from back to front with a tongue-scraper device) and tooth brushing, is said to help remove toxins that accumulate in your mouth overnight from your body's metabolic processes. Not only do these techniques leave your mouth feeling fresher, they can also boost your health and wellbeing.

4 Activate your digestion

There's a good reason why yogis start their day with a cup of warm water and lemon. Warm water acts on the intestinal tract, helping to stimulate the digestion and kickstart your metabolism in the morning. Meanwhile, the slice of fresh lemon or squeeze of juice helps reduce inflammation in the body and provides valuable vitamins to keep you well. Try making the swap from your regular cuppa tomorrow and see if you notice the difference.

5 Bathe well

Bathing or showering in the morning isn't just a practical way to freshen up for the day ahead. Yogis believe it energises your body, clears your mind and brings a sense of holiness to your day. If you have time – perhaps at the weekend – begin by massaging your body and scalp with warm oil (try coconut or sesame oil). This practice is known as abhyanga and boosts your circulation and energy while aiding detoxification, lowering stress and easing muscle tension. Follow your massage with a mindful shower or bath, spending a few minutes enjoying the refreshing sensations and sounds of the water as you wash.

6 Stretch yourself

Now is the perfect time to start your morning yoga routine. It will gently wake up your body and mind, remove sluggishness, lift your mood, ignite your digestive fire and bring focus for the day. Listen to your body and choose a selection of yoga poses (p38) or sequences (p102) to suit how you feel today, mentally and physically. If you have time, follow up your physical practice with some Pranayama (breathing exercises, p118) and/or meditation (p122) to help set your intention and ground yourself for the day ahead.

7 Breakfast wisely

We all know the expression 'breakfast like a king' but yogis believe you should always eat a light, healthy breakfast. This avoids straining your digestive fire which only comes into full force in the middle of the day when kapha time has ended. It's always best to leave two hours between eating a meal and doing yoga so stick to just warm water and lemon or herbal tea before your morning practice, and then enjoy breakfast after you finish when your appetite will be strong. Opt for healthy choices such as fruit, muesli, grain porridges or vegetable juices.

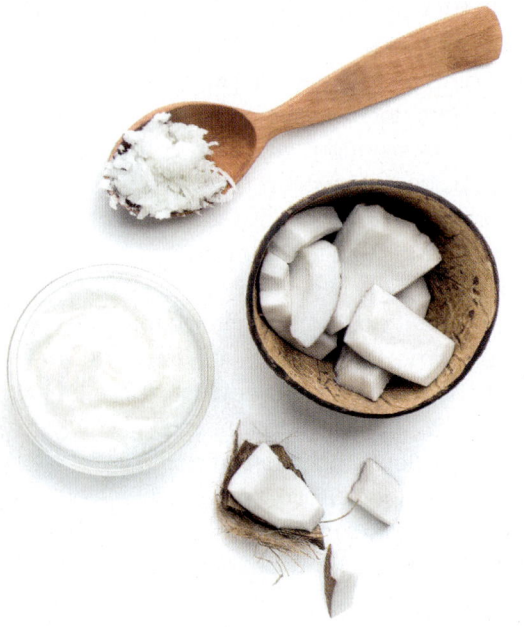

Morning rituals

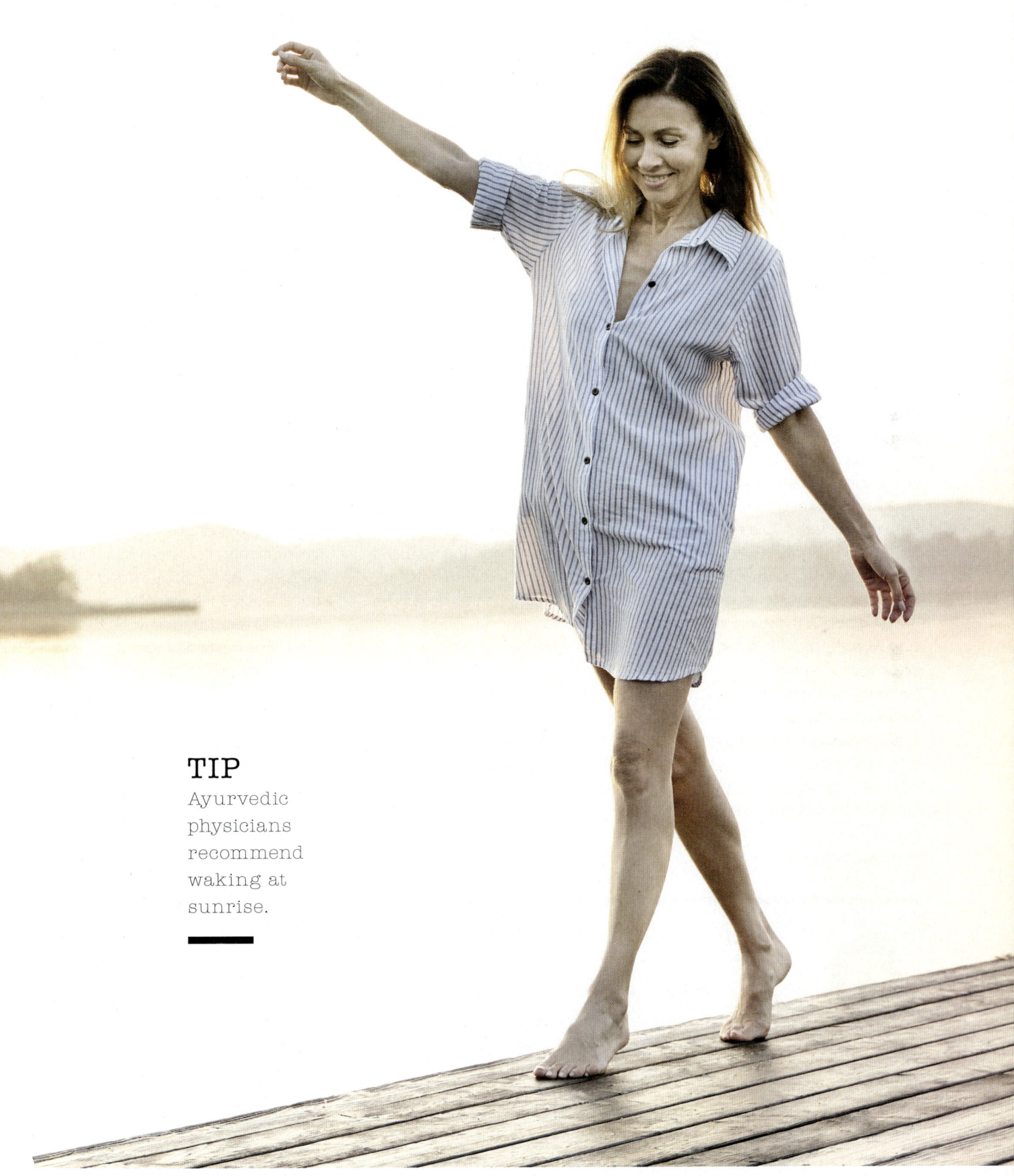

TIP
Ayurvedic physicians recommend waking at sunrise.

Biographies

MEET THE EXPERTS

We hope you've enjoyed discovering the joys of morning yoga! Meet the expert instructors who have contributed to this book

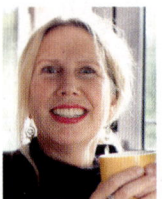

Laura Gate-Eastley
Yoga sequences (page 108)

Laura has been teaching yoga for 20 years after falling in love with the way the practice kept her grounded during her previous life in the music industry. For many years, a daily Ashtanga practice sustained her. In addition to assisting her teachers at Triyoga in London, Laura trained with Brian Cooper and Nawajyoti at Union Yoga in Edinburgh. She added to the 200hr Yoga Alliance certification with Vinyasa flow training with Shiva Rea, annual retreats with her teacher Clive Sheridan and workshops with other inspirational teachers. In 2020, Laura completed her Meditation Teacher Training with Cyndi Lee and Restorative yoga training with Adelene Cheong. She has now fully embraced her own online teaching. For Laura's class schedule and more information *visit lauralotus.co.uk.*

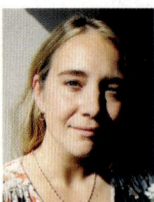

Hanna-Jade Browne
Breathe into being (page 118)

Hanna-Jade has dedicated 10 years to studying, practising and sharing natural healing. After leaving the music industry, she spent four years studying bio-medicine, naturopathy and nutrition, before travelling to India where she met her spiritual teacher who introduced her to rebirthing and breathwork. Hanna-Jade trained in traditional Hatha yoga (200 hours) and ayurvedic studies in the Himalayas, continuing to live and serve at the ashram. Later, she qualified as a therapeutic practitioner in integrative breathwork with schools including Rebirthing, Transformational Breath and Bio-dynamic Breathwork & Trauma Release System, plus sound healing with the Acutonics system and is a Reiki master. Hanna-Jade is founder of Embodhi Breath and offers classes and workshops worldwide. *Visit embodhibreath.life.*

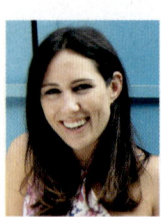

Ali Roff Farrar
Mindful mornings (page 122)

Ali is a yoga teacher, mindfulness expert, wellness editor, author, and Wellness Director at *Psychologies* magazine. Her debut book *The Wellfulness Project* (Aster) is out now. Ali is passionate about combining the western sciences of psychology, neuroscience and coaching with the eastern philosophies of meditation, mindfulness and yoga to cultivate true wellness of body and mind. In addition to holding a BSc Hons degree in Psychology, Ali is a qualified 200hr Yoga Alliance Certified teacher and soon to qualify as a mindfulness teacher for stress and chronic pain. Ali also runs a yoga, mindfulness and fitness retreat and brunch company with her husband. Together, they are founders of online wellness platform Wellfulness (mywellfulness.com). For more information about Ali, *visit aliroff.com.*

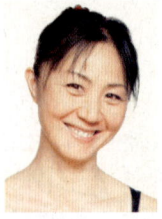

Aki Omori
Yoga instruction

Aki is a yoga teacher with more than 20 years' experience. She is also a leading Restorative yoga expert, somatic movement therapist and educator. Aki practised yoga for many years with Clive Sheridan, Donna Farhi and Erich Schiffmann. She teaches regular classes at Triyoga in London as well as providing private yoga tuition, online classes, teacher training, workshops and international retreats. For more information and details of Aki's classes, *visit akiomori.blogspot.com.*

Props
+ Yoga Matters (yogamatters.com)
+ Manduka (manduka.com)
+ Gaiam (gaiam.co.uk)

Online yoga
+ Laura Gate-Eastley (bookwhen.com/lauralotus)
+ Triyoga (Triyoga.co.uk)
+ Re:Mind Studio (tv.remindstudio.com)

Find a teacher
+ British Wheel of Yoga (bwy.org.uk)
+ Yoga Alliance (yogaalliance.co.uk)